The Limits of Statins: Uncovering Treatment Options for Heart Valve Disease

Brad

Table of Contents

Chapter 1: Introduction

1.1 Overview

1.1.1 The Cardiac Valves

The human heart beats over 3 billion times during an average lifespan, continuously delivering oxygenated blood to the body and deoxygenated blood to the lungs. The closed circulatory system of humans and mammals requires unidirectional blood flow in order to ensure delivery of an appropriate amount of oxygen and nutrients. Heart valves are essential structures for maintaining this unidirectional blood flow by opening and closing at appropriate times throughout the cardiac cycle. Mammals and birds have 4 heart valves: the tricuspid, the pulmonic, the aortic (AoV) and the mitral. The atrioventricular valves (tricuspid and mitral) open to allow blood to flow from the atria into the ventricles, while the semilunar valves (pulmonic and AoV) open to allow blood to flow into pulmonic artery and aorta respectively [1]. Although the function of each valve is similar, their macro-structures are diverse. The aortic and pulmonic valves are composed of three leaflets, termed cusps, and contain integrated internal supporting structures [2]. The tricuspid valve similarly possesses three leaflets but utilizes external tendonous support structures called chordae tendineae, which connect the ventricular side of the leaflets to the papillary muscles of the heart and prevent inversion of the valve leaflets during the cardiac cycle.

1

The supporting structures of the mitral valve are similar, but this left-sided valve has only two leaflets [3, 4].

The AoV is the focus of this dissertation, and therefore the structure and function of this particular valve will be outlined in more detail. As described, the AoV is composed of three cusps which are classified according to their relationship to the coronary arteries, which connect to the aorta just above the plane of the valve. The cusps directly adjacent to the coronaries are termed the left coronary (L/C) and right coronary (R/C) cusps respectively, while the remaining cusp is the noncoronary (N/C) [5, 6]. These cusps experience a constant variety of mechanical stresses as they open and close during the cardiac cycle [7]. During systole as the heart contracts to pump blood out to the body, the AoV must open fully to allow for maximum flow, while during diastole, the cusps remain tightly closed to prevent regurgitation of blood into the left ventricle. This pattern creates a set of conditions in which different regions of the AoV cusps experience a range of unevenly distributed mechanical forces including oscillatory shear, laminar shear, pressure, and stretch, all at different points in the cycle [5, 8].

1.1.2 Valve Extracellular Matrix

To withstand these forces and provide proper AoV function, each cusp is densely packed with three layers of extracellular matrix (ECM) proteins which are organized in a side-specific manner to support the required biomechanical functions throughout the cardiac cycle [9]. The fibrosa is present on the aortic side of each cusp and is composed mainly of collagens. While a variety of collagens are present, the most abundant are the fibrillar collagen types I and III [10, 11] which form tightly packed collagen bundles that orient parallel to the valve edge. This arrangement provides tensile strength to the cusp while still allowing for stretch. The spongiosa is adjacent to the fibrosa and consists of a variety of proteoglycans and glycosaminoglycans including hyaluronic acid, chondroitin sulfates such as versican, and decorin [12]. These ECM components function to bind water molecules and facilitate compression, allowing the valve to absorb energy from high-pressure blood flow. The third ECM layer is present on the ventricular side of each AoV cusp and primarily includes elastin, which provide elasticity to allow the cusp to return to its native conformation between cardiac cycles [13]. The precise organization and composition of each of these three layers is extremely important for proper development and biomechanical function of the AoV, and conservation of this same ECM arrangement is also necessary for function of the other three cardiac valves (Fig. 1) [2, 14].

1.1.3 Valve Cell Populations

In addition to the ECM, the AoV, similar to the other cardiac valves, includes dynamic cell populations that collectively maintain homeostasis and organization of these structural proteins. The most abundant cell population in the AoV are the valve interstitial cells (VICs), which are found throughout all three layers of the ECM. Although this population is heterogenous based on molecular profiles and embryonic origins [15, 16], a common feature is their role in regulating the ECM components of the valve through their expression and production of collagens, proteoglycans and elastins, as well as enzymes which degrade or organize these ECM components as part of the physiological maintenance process [17, 18]. Various studies have shown the ability of the VICs to utilize cell-cell as well as cell-ECM signaling in order to adapt appropriately to any environmental changes [19-21], but details about these exact mechanisms are still an active area of investigation.

A second prominent cell type are valve endothelial cells (VECs) that form a continuous single cell layer over the lining of each AoV cusp. By extending long cytoplasmic projections and forming impermeable tight junctions with neighboring cells, the VECs are able to create a protective layer which shields the inner VICs and ECM from the external environment [14, 22, 23]. However, the VECs play a role far beyond that of a barrier. Many groups have demonstrated the importance of the VEC population in establishing and regulating AoV signaling pathways [24-26]. Due to their positioning, the VECs function as an interface between the surrounding environment and the inner VICs and ECM by using mechanosensitive surface glycoproteins to detect changes in mechanical stresses [22, 27-29].

A recent study utilizing single-cell RNA-seq has shown that the VECs are heterogeneous and include three distinct subpopulations which express transcripts associated with the mechanical forces they experience based on their position on the AoV cusp. VECs expressing classical endothelial markers such as von Willebrand Factor (vWF) are located on both the fibrosa and ventricularis side of each cusp. The second subset of VECs expresses transcripts involved in lymph vessel development and is located away from pulsatile blood flow. A third transcriptionally distinct group is located in regions of high mechanical stress, particularly at the coaptation point at the tip of the valve which experiences high shear stress during systole and high pressure during diastole. These coaptation-VECs express high levels of cytoskeletal organization transcripts.

This and other studies proving region-specific roles of endothelial cells indicate the importance of VEC mechanosensing in establishing phenotypes and signaling in the AoV [30, 31]. The VECs signal to VICs through both paracrine signals and direct mechanical transmission through focal adhesion complexes [23, 24, 32, 33]. The VICs then work to modify the ECM by producing additional matrix proteins, degrading existing matrix, or synthesizing ECM-organizing enzymes [17, 18]. These relationships create a signaling network which connects the valve environment, VECs, VICs, and ECM. However, the exact signaling pathways that connect mechanosensitive responses in VECs to active remodeling of the ECM by VICs are still not well understood.

Based on current knowledge in the field, the remaining cells in the AoV have been broadly grouped into two categories: immune cells and melanocytes. It has been well established that immune cells are present within the valve cusp [30, 34, 35]. Common immune cell types include CD45-positive bone marrow derived cells and CCR2-positive macrophage, but there are a wide variety of markers which correspond with hematopoietic origin and stage of differentiation [30, 34]. Although the role and function of these cells is still being elucidated, studies from our group have shown that these cells are recruited from the bone marrow and take up residence in the AoV cusp, as their numbers increase with age [34, 36], and they may play a role in normal valve homeostasis [35]. The role of melanocytes in the AoV is less clear, although it is known that their abundance varies by species and individual. It has been hypothesized that they also possess an immunological function [37, 38], and other studies have shown a potential relationship between melanocytes and valve tissue stiffness [39, 40].

1.2.1 Embryonic Development

Cardiac valve development is an organized process which begins around embryonic day (e) 9.5 in the mouse and e31 in the human [41, 42]. AoV development begins in the heart tube with the formation of endocardial cushions. These cushions are surrounded by a layer of endothelial cells and contain the cardiac jelly, a proteoglycan-rich ECM produced by the adjacent myocardium [6, 16, 43]. While the distal outflow tract cushions go on to develop the aorticopulmonary septum, a subset of endothelial cells in the proximal outflow tract cushion undergo endothelial-to-mesenchymal transition (endMT), during which they detach from the endothelial layer and proliferate and migrate into the cardiac jelly to form the valve precursor cell pool [6, 43-45]. The endMT process is driven by complex coordinated interactions of signaling pathways including Tgfβ, Wnt, Vegf, Nfatc1, BMP, Sox9 and Notch [16, 43, 46, 47]. These signals allow the VECs to detach and migrate away from the endocardium while taking on a new cellular identity and phenotype in response [48, 49].

Although the process of endMT is critically important for generating the VIC precursors in the developing AoV, it has been well-established that additional cell lineages, including cardiac neural crest and secondary heart field (SHF), add to this population [15, 50-52]. The exact function of these contributions is still an active area of study, but it is known that the distinct migration patterns result in cusp-specific differences that may have important developmental consequences. The L/C and R/C AoV cusps contain mainly endMT-derived cells with some neural crest contribution [16, 53, 54], while the N/C cusp contains a greater abundance of SHF-derived cells [55, 56].

As the proximal endocardial cushion forms and expands, a process of excavation and sculpting begins. A combination of programmed cell death and selective endothelial growth and proliferation along the arterial edge of the cushion allows for shaping of the typical elongated valve cusp [6]. During this time, the mesenchymal cell population inside the cushion moves toward a differentiated phenotype, taking on markers of active VICs, including smooth muscle alpha actin (α-SMA). These activated VICs continue to proliferate and remodel the cardiac jelly into a more mature ECM containing collagens, proteoglycans, and elastins which will continue to stratify into layers throughout development and maturation [6, 53, 57].

1.2.2 Postnatal Growth and Adult Maintenance

After birth, changes in blood flow patterns allow for further shaping of the valve cusps through a less-studied process involving VIC phenotypes and continuing ECM remodeling and stratification [6, 57]. Proliferation rates of valve cells reach their peak at murine postnatal day (PND) 2 (Nordquist, data not shown), and the elongation and remodeling process continues until the AoV cusps have reached a mature morphology by approximately PND 7. At this point, VICs begin to downregulate markers of activation and take on a more quiescent phenotype where ECM remodeling and production are relatively minimal and cell turnover is low. In the absence of any perturbations, the mature valve will maintain this quiescent state throughout adulthood [58, 59]. Exact rates of cell and ECM turnover during adult valve homeostasis are relatively understudied, but proliferation is generally thought to be occurring in less than 1% of valve cells at any given time, and the overall cell density in the valve decreases throughout life [57, 60]. Although it is clear that postnatal valve development and adult valve maintenance are characterized by different proliferation rates, ECM conditions, and signaling mechanisms, the key changes in molecular profiles which promote these different states have not yet been elucidated.

1.3 Valve Disease

1.3.1 Overview

When either valve development or the homeostatic maintenance of the valve is disrupted, disease can result. The spectrum of valve disease ranges from congenital malformations such as bicuspid aortic valve (BAV) to acquired valve disease which can present as a wide variety of phenotypes. Regardless of how disease presents, the outcome of valve disease is an overall morphological change resulting in the inability of the valve to correctly preserve unidirectional blood flow [3]. Although all four cardiac valves are known to develop disease, the aortic valve is most commonly affected [61], likely due to the higher pressures and shear force the valve experiences as blood flows from the left ventricle into the aorta. AoV disease overall represents a significant public health burden, with the prevalence at over 2.5% in the US alone [62]. These patients experience symptoms that can affect quality of life, such as shortness of breath, fainting, and chest pain. If untreated, valve disease can ultimately lead to heart failure [3].

1.3.2 Risk Factors

While congenital valve diseases are often due to genetic factors, the molecular etiology of acquired valve disease is not as well understood. However, it is clear that certain risk factors can contribute to the likelihood and severity of valve disease. These can include cigarette smoking, high blood pressure, cholesterol imbalance, and metabolic factors including diabetes [63, 64]. However, the most prominent risk factor for the development of valve disease is age. More than 10% of the population over age 80 experiences valve disease [65]. The precise reason for the increase in valve disease incidence with age is still an area of investigation, although studies have shown age-related changes in both the cell and matrix components of the AoV, which may be linked to disease development [60, 66, 67].

1.3.3 Valve Endothelial Cell Damage and Dysfunction

Previous work from our group and others has shown that the molecular and physical properties of VECs in particular experience age-related changes. Functionally, VECs in aging valves produce less nitric oxide (NO), an important signal mediator in VEC to VIC communication. Additionally, aging valves tend to have a lower overall number of VECs which become spaced farther apart on the surface of each cusp. This age-related change in morphology allows the endothelial barrier to become more permeable to circulating molecules [16, 28, 60].

Due to these age-related changes, the VEC population is an important factor in the development of both acquired and congenital valve diseases. Recently, a consensus in the field has been reached that places VEC dysfunction and injury as the primary initiating factor for disease development [68-72]. Following this disruption of the VEC barrier, inflammatory cells, lipids, or calcium deposits accumulate at the most permeable segments and begin to infiltrate the valve cusp, triggering a cascade of events which result in the alteration of ECM production by the VICs and ultimately a diseased valve morphology [22, 68, 73, 74]. The evidence for this theory comes from studies of diseased human valves displaying damaged VECs and an overall lack of endothelial integrity [75] as well as murine models of endothelial-specific genetic manipulation, injury, or dysfunction resulting in valve disease [26, 58, 76].

While damage to the VEC barrier and risk factor infiltration clearly contribute to disease pathogenesis, disturbed VEC-VIC communication likely plays a role as well. It is well established that during the disease process, VICs exit their healthy quiescent phase and take on an "activated" state during which they express markers such as α-SMA and begin to remodel the ECM in a process similar to valve development. However, *in vitro* studies have demonstrated that the activation of VICs change according to the presence or absence of VECs, and this dependence is based on chemical and physical signaling from VECs. Signaling from VECs is essential for maintaining VIC and overall valve homeostasis, indicating that a disruption of this communication may lead to pathological VIC activation and ECM remodeling [25, 26, 33, 77]. Therefore, preservation of VEC function and the endothelial barrier are critical for maintaining healthy valve structure and preventing development of disease.

1.4 Treatment and Management of Valve Disease

1.4.1   Current Treatment Options

Although the prevalence of valve disease is high and expected to increase over the coming decade [78], current treatment options remain limited. Symptom and risk factor treatment can be beneficial in the early stages of valve disease, while surgical repair or replacement remains the only true treatment for advanced valve disease [79, 80]. One limited therapeutic option to decrease risk factors is oral statin therapy to correct cholesterol imbalance. Studies on patients receiving this type of treatment report declining low-density lipoprotein (LDL) levels but ultimately little improvement in overall valve function [15, 81-84]. Other pharmaceutical alternatives include medications to lower blood pressure and introduce blood thinners. Lifestyle changes can also have an impact on risk factor levels and therefore valve disease development [80].

Because so few pharmaceutical treatments are available, surgery remains the standard protocol for valve disease that has progressed [79, 80]. For certain cases of milder valve disease, repair of existing valve cusps is possible and allows the majority of the native valve structure to be preserved. Some cases of disease, especially in high risk or elderly patients, can also be treated with balloon valvuloplasty procedures, which use minimally invasive techniques to widen a narrowed valve opening [85, 86]. However, these methods are limited and often act as shorter-term solutions [86, 87], as more advanced disease often requires total valve replacement.

Surgical replacement is an open-heart procedure where the diseased valve is removed and completely replaced by a prosthetic or bioprosthetic valve, while the newer method of transcatheter aortic valve replacement (TAVR) is less invasive and involves insertion of the replacement valve directly into the existing diseased valve structure [80]. Although these surgical procedures are often successful in treating valve disease, they are not without faults. There is always risk associated with surgery, especially for older patients or patients with preexisting conditions who may be ineligible for major procedures.

Additionally, mechanical valves increase the likelihood of blood clots and so require anticoagulation therapy, while bioprosthetic valves (usually made from bovine or porcine tissue) have a limited longevity and often require repeat surgery in the patient's lifetime [88, 89].

1.4.2 *Endogenous Self-Repair*

While advances in existing therapies and surgical technologies have been beneficial, there remains a critical lack of treatment options for valve disease patients. One new area of exploration in treatment for valve disease is the promotion of endogenous self-repair, with cell proliferation acting as a key component. This idea has been well-studied in other fields such as myocardial and vascular biology but remains a fairly novel area of research in the valve field.

In exploring how to repair damaged heart muscle following an injury such as myocardial infarction, many groups have examined the response of the myocardium and its ability to heal [90-93]. These studies have shown that while the adult mammalian heart has extremely limited regenerative capacity, during a window of developmental time shortly after birth the heart is able to functionally repair damage on its own by upregulating proliferation of existing un-damaged cardiomyocytes [94, 95]. An analogous process occurs in the zebrafish myocardium after injury, but zebrafish maintain the capacity to self-repair beyond a developmental window and into adulthood [96, 97]. Similarly, it has been shown that proliferation of existing local cells is responsible for the restoration of the endothelial lining of the aorta, which often becomes damaged over time in a manner similar to the AoV. However, distinct from the mammalian myocardium, the aortic vasculature in mammals appears to retain this self-repair capacity even into adult stages [98]. The hope for these lines of experimentation is to discover the factors which promote this repair in order to pharmaceutically upregulate the repair process to prevent disease development or progression.

Existing work in this area in the valves is relatively limited, but very recent studies have confirmed that valvular regeneration is possible in an adult zebrafish model. These experiments utilized a chemogenetic model to ablate the VIC population of the valve and subsequently observe the regeneration process. It was seen that new cells in the regenerated valve resulted from a combination of proliferation of endogenous valve cells and localization of kidney marrow cells to the valve site [99, 100]. A much earlier *ex vivo* study of the repair of a porcine valve after endothelial injury also confirms the ability of valve cells to respond to an injury in a manner consistent with repair and regeneration [101]. Future studies elucidating the mechanisms behind valvular self-repair in different model systems will be needed in order to fully understand the process and work towards development of non-surgical therapies.

1.5 Summary and Closing

1.5.1   Summary

The AoV contains abundant and stratified ECM in addition to two prominent cell types, VICs and VECs. Together, these components form an extremely important element of the cardiovascular system. Through a coordinated process, the AoV begins as endocardial cushions and eventually elongates and develops into a valve structure with the exact biomechanical properties necessary to preserve unidirectional blood flow.

Unfortunately, valve disease can occur as a result of a congenital malformation or as an acquired disease. Of the risk factors that may increase the likelihood of valve disease development, aging is the most prominent. Age-related changes in VEC function have been observed and may contribute to disease development, as studies have shown that VEC damage or injury is a primary factor in the initiation of valve disease. Current therapies are limited, and patients with symptomatic valve disease almost always require surgical intervention as disease progresses. However, research in the field of regeneration of the valves has recently provided a promising window into the potential for upregulation of self-repair mechanisms as a therapeutic treatment for valve disease which could improve patient quality of life and outcomes.

1.5.2 Closing

The goal of the work included in the following chapters of this dissertation is to advance the growing body of knowledge surrounding valve damage and endogenous repair mechanisms with the hope that this data will add to our understanding of valve disease development and contribute to non-surgical patient treatment in the future. The initial focus of these studies, detailed in Chapter 2, was to examine potential developmental mechanisms which could be applied to promote repair or regeneration in adult stages. This line of research led to the experiments in Chapter 3, which involve the adaptation of an *in vivo* murine valve injury model to further examine the overall valve response to endothelial damage and explore endogenous repair mechanisms. The studies have generated compelling results with the potential for future in-depth studies which are described in corresponding chapters.

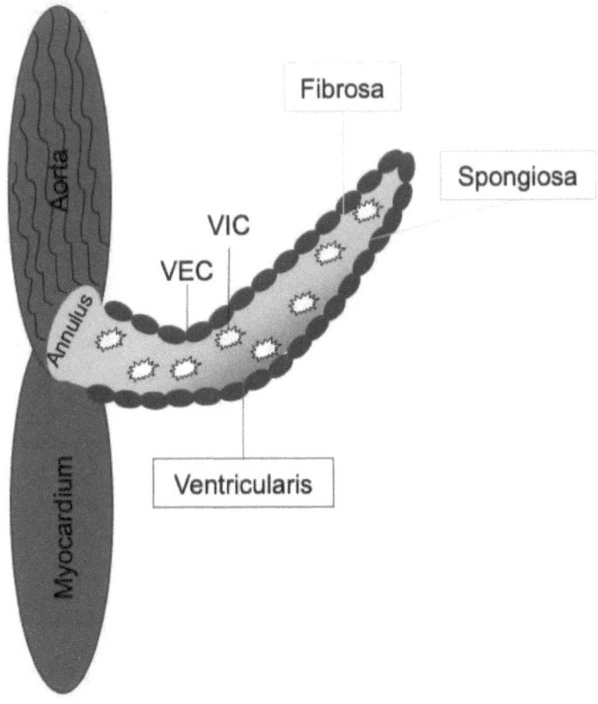

Figure 1: Cross Section of the Aortic Valve Cusp.

The AoV cusp contains three distinct ECM layers, the fibrosa (yellow), spongiosa (blue), and ventricularis (grey). The two main cell types in the AoV are the VICs (white) and VECs (gray). The fibrous annulus connects the valve cusp to the larger structure of the heart.

Chapter 2: Postnatal and Adult Aortic Heart Valves Have Distinctive Transcriptional Profiles Associated with Valve Tissue Growth and Maintenance Respectively[1]

2.1 Introduction

The average heart beats over a billion times during one lifespan to continuously provide blood to every part of the body. Crucial to this task are the four heart valves (aortic, pulmonic, tricuspid and mitral), that function to maintain the unidirectional flow of oxygenated and unoxygenated blood. Distinct from the cardiac muscle, the mature valve leaflets are highly organized structures comprised of three layers of extracellular matrix (ECM) components including collagens, proteoglycans, and elastin [2]. Formation and maintenance of the valve ECM is mediated by a heterogeneous population of valve interstitial cells (VICs) that are fibroblast-like in phenotype [102]. Surrounding the VICs and ECM is a single layer of valve endothelial cells (VECs) that physically protect the valve from external stimuli, and molecularly communicate with underlying VICs to regulate homeostasis of the ECM [25, 26, 60]. The complex relationship between valve cell populations and the ECM is critical for establishing and maintaining structure-function

[1] Adapted from Nordquist E, LaHaye S, Nagel C, Lincoln, J. "Postnatal and Adult Aortic Valves Have Distinct Transcriptional Profiles Associated with Valve Tissue Growth and Maintenance Respectively." *Frontiers in Cardiovascular Medicine*, April 2018.

Author contributions: experimental data was collected by EN, and RNA-seq performed and analyzed by CN. Additional analysis of RNA-seq data was undertaken by SL. EN and JL generated the manuscript with input from SL.

relationships throughout life. This relationship begins during embryonic development, as mesenchymal precursor cells in the endocardial cushions transition towards an activated VIC phenotype and degrade primitive ECM within the cushions while secreting more diverse ECM components. Elongation and remodeling of the immature valve structures continues for a short time during the postnatal period, until around postnatal day 10 in the mouse when the ECM components are more defined. Once valve formation is complete, VICs convert to a quiescent phenotype and in the absence of disease, maintain physiological turnover of the ECM to provide efficient function throughout life (reviewed [72, 102]). While the regulation of valve development is well established, the mechanisms that regulate postnatal valve growth and remodeling, as well as adult homeostasis are poorly understood. Despite constant mechanical demand on the valve leaflets, turnover of valve cell populations in adult valves is relatively low [60]. Therefore, it remains unclear how structure-function relationships are maintained throughout life in healthy individuals, yet dysregulation of these relationships likely underlies the onset and progression of valve dysfunction and disease.

Heart valve disease is a growing public health problem that can affect both adult and pediatric patients. Significant defects during embryonic valve development lead to congenital malformations which compromise the typical structure of the valve, leading to reduced ability to function correctly (reviewed [103]). Distinct from valve disease present at birth, pathology can also be acquired and is most prevalent in the aging population, with up to 13% of people aged over 75 affected [104]. It is well known that aging increases the onset of valve diseases including calcification or myxomatous degeneration, and this is likely attributed to decades of exposure to risk factors including hypercholesterolemia, tobacco-use, hypertension and overall wear-and-tear. In young adults, valve disease is less prevalent, possibly resulting from the fact that the healthy valve is able to maintain homeostasis by repairing small amounts of damage that occur due to normal mechanical stress, which has been shown in non-valvular cardiac tissues [94] . Many believe that with age, the valve loses this ability to 'self-repair', resulting in significant damage, injury, or loss to the valve cell populations, and it has been shown that altered VEC function leads to VIC-mediated dysregulation of ECM homeostasis [26, 60, 72]. Currently, the only effective treatment for valve disease is surgical repair or replacement, resulting in over 90,000 valve replacement surgeries performed in the US each year [105]. Surgical treatment comes with many complications including the need for repeat surgeries due to low valve durability and high thrombogenicity, in addition to the large personal and societal economic burdens [106]. Therefore, there is a critical need for the development of alternate therapeutics.

A promising therapeutic area is emerging in the field of regenerative medicine. Common to both congenital and age-related valve disease is the damage and consequent loss of healthy cell populations alongside the development of pathological cell populations which are unable to preserve the correct structure of the valve and therefore lead to functional failure [48]. The therapeutic ability to replenish the lost population of healthy cells would allow for correction of ECM deposition, leading to recovery of structure and therefore function of the valve. The field of cardiac regeneration has recently made significant advances in elucidating the molecular mechanisms of regeneration, although these studies have mainly focused on the myocardium, leaving a need for more investigation into the valve. In the myocardium, several key studies in murine models have shown that the neonatal heart has remarkable regenerative capacity during the first week of life, and this regenerative potential corresponds with endogenous cardiomyocyte proliferation, which drastically decreases after postnatal day 7 [107-109]. Further investigation has led to the discovery of specific influential regulators of this innate regeneration program, which include pathways such as Nrg1-ErbB [90] and Hippo signaling [110], as well alterations in matrix rigidity due to ECM components such as Agrin [93]. The ability to recapitulate these neonatal proliferation programs in adult mammalian hearts has proven to be successful in promoting myocardial regeneration after injury and in disease models [93, 111]. Considerably less is known about the regenerative capacity of the heart valves. Current studies indicate there may be a population of progenitor-like VECs that have the ability to undergo 'developmental-like' endothelial to mesenchymal transition (endMT) in response to pathophysiologic conditions in order to replenish diseased or damaged VICs [48]. There is also evidence that hematopoietic-derived CD45-positive cells contribute to valve maintenance as cells are lost or damaged at a homeostatic level [36]. However, knowledge is still lacking regarding molecular mechanisms of valve cell proliferation or regeneration potential.

The goal of the current study is to initiate discovery of potential mechanisms that may promote growth or replenishment of functional cell populations in the adult valve. To do this, we used RNA-seq analysis to explore differential molecular profiles between postnatal and adult valve cell populations. This analysis will help define potential regeneration indicators that in the future might be reintroduced in diseased or aging adult valves to increase their self-repair capacity and improve structure-function relationships. Our study has defined transcriptional differences between postnatal day 2 (PND2) and adult (4 months) aortic valves and identified significant changes in key biological functions related to cell proliferation, extracellular matrix, and defense response that may be important for determining the regenerative capacity of the valve to aid in the future development of alternative therapeutics.

2.2 Materials and Methods

2.2.1 Mice

C57BL/6J mice were fed regular chow mix and housed in a controlled environment with 12-hour light/dark cycles at 21°C and 23% humidity and water ad libitum. Animals were euthanized by CO_2 exposure followed by secondary euthanasia by cervical dislocation (adult mice) or decapitation (pups). All animal procedures were approved by The Research Institute at Nationwide Children's Hospital Institutional Animal Care and Use Committee (Protocol # AR13-00054).

2.2.2 Tissue Preparation

Hearts were collected from postnatal day 2 (PND2) and 4 month old *C57BL/6J* mice and fixed in 4% paraformaldehyde/1xPBS overnight at 4°C. For paraffin sections, tissue was embedded in paraffin wax and sectioned at 10μm. Paraffin was removed in xylenes, and tissue sections were re-hydrated through a graded ethanol series and rinsed in 1xPBS as previously described [53]. Tissue sections containing aortic valves were then subjected to Movat's Pentachrome staining, EdU staining, or immunohistochemistry/immunofluorescence (see below for details). For cryo sections, tissue was embedded in OCT and frozen, then sectioned at 7μm. Prior to staining, tissue was permeabilized using 0.1% triton-X 100 in 1xPBS and then subjected to immunofluorescence staining.

2.2.3 Immunohistochemistry/Immunofluorescence

Whole hearts from PND2 and 4 month old *C57BL6J* mice were collected and prepared according to above methods. Movat's Pentachrome staining was performed on paraffin tissue sections at each time point according to the manufacturer's instructions (Russel Movat, American MasterTech, #KTRMP), then mounted using VectaMount Permanent Mounting Medium (Vector Laboratories, H-5000). For antibody detection, fixed paraffin tissue sections were subjected to antigen retrieval by boiling for 10 minutes in unmasking solution (Vector Laboratories), and both cryo and paraffin sections were subjected to blocking for 1 hour at room temperature (1% BSA, 1% cold water fish skin gelatin, 0.1% Tween-20/PBS) as described [112]. Tissue sections were then incubated overnight at 4°C or 1 hour at room temperature with primary antibodies against Mmp3 (rabbit, 1:100 paraffin, Abcam ab53015), Nid2 (rabbit, 1:200 cryo, Abcam ab14513), Ptgs2 (Rabbit, 1:100 paraffin, Cell Signaling 12282), and Rarres2 (Mouse, 1:100 paraffin, Santa Cruz sc-373797). For immunofluorescent primary antibody detection of Mmp3, Nid2, and Ptgs2, sections were incubated for 1 hour at room temperature with Donkey anti-rabbit or Goat anti-rabbit Alexa-Fluor IgG secondary antibodies (1:500) (LifeTechnologies), then mounted in Vectashield anti-fade medium with DAPI (Vector Laboratories) to detect cell nuclei. For DAB staining of Rarres2, sections were stained using Mouse and Rabbit Specific HRP/DAB (ABC) Detection IHC kit (Abcam, ab64264), counterstained with hematoxylin (Vector Laboratories, H-3404), and mounted using VectaMount Permanent mounting medium (Vector Laboratories, H-5000). Images were visualized using an Olympus BX51 microscope and captured using an Olympus DP71 camera and CellSens software. Image brightness and contrast were edited using Adobe Photoshop CC.

2.2.4 EdU Staining and Quantification

PND2 and 4 month old *C57BL/6J* mice were injected subcutaneously with 10μg/g body weight EdU (Invitrogen) dissolved in 1xPBS. 24 hours later, mice were sacrificed and hearts were collected and prepared according to above methods. Fixed tissue sections were blocked for 1 hour at room temperature (1% BSA, 0.1% Cold water fish skin gelatin, 0.1% Tween 20 in PBS with 0.05% NaN_3), followed by use of Click-it EdU Kit (Invitrogen) to detect presence of EdU according to the manufacturer's instructions. Sections were then mounted in Vectashield anti-fade medium with DAPI (Vector Laboratories) to detect cell nuclei. The total number of cell nuclei in one leaflet were counted using ImageJ cell counter. Number of EdU-positive cells were then counted and calculated as a percentage of total cells. Statistical analysis was performed in GraphPad Prism 7.0a.

2.2.5 Aortic Valve Isolation and RNA-Sequencing

Aortic valves from wild type PND2 and 4 month old *C57BL/6J* mice were isolated with minimal myocardial contamination and immediately flash frozen in liquid nitrogen.

Frozen samples were sent to Ocean Ridge Biosciences LLC (Palm Gardens Beach, FL), where RNA isolation and sequencing was performed as follows. Total RNA was extracted using the TRI Reagent® (Molecular Research Center; Part #: TR118) method, and isolated RNA was quantified using chip-based capillary electrophoresis (Agilent 2100 Bioanalyzer Pico Chip). RNA was digested with RNase free DNase I (Epicentre; Part # D9905K) and purified through minElute columns (Qiagen; Part #: 74204). Final RNA samples were quantified by O.D. measurement and re-quantified using chip-based capillary electrophoresis. Amplified cDNA libraries were prepared from 200 nanograms on DNA-free total RNA using TruSeq Stranded Total mRNA Library Prep Kit LT (Illumina Inc.; Part #s: RS-122-2101 and RS-122-2102). Chip-based capillary electrophoresis was used to assess quality and size distribution of the libraries. KAPA Library Quantification Kit (Kapa Biosystems, Boston, MA) was used to quantify the libraries. Libraries were pooled at equimolar concentrations and were clustered on an Illumina cBot cluster station. Clustering was performed with the HiSeq PE cluster kit v4 and sequenced on an Illumina HiSeq Flow Cell v4 with 50 nt paired-end reads plus dual index reads using the Illumina HiSeq SBS Kit v4. An average of approximately 48.3 million passed-filter 50 nucleotide paired-end reads were obtained per sample (24.1M per direction).

Raw FASTQs were split into files containing 4,000,000 reads and checked for quality using the FASTX-Toolkit. The reads were filtered (removing sequences that did not pass Illumina's quality filter) and trimmed based on the quality results (3 nucleotides at the left end of the R1 reads and 1 nt at the left end of the R2 reads). Sequence alignment was performed using TopHat v2.1.0 to the mm10 genome. BAM files were merged on a per sample. Exon and gene level counting were performed using the easyRNASeq version 2.4.7 package. A binary annotation file, built using the annotation file generation function of EasyRNASeq, was used for this analysis; the Ensembl release 83 GTF file was used as input. Annotation was performed using a Gene Transfer Format (GTF) annotation file for Mus musculus, which was downloaded on February 11, 2016 and contains the current Ensembl Mouse release 83. Filtering of the RPKM values was performed to retain a list of genes with a minimum of approximately 50 mapped reads in 25% or more samples. The threshold of 50 mapped reads is considered the Reliable Quantification Threshold, as the reads per kilobase million (RPKM) values for a gene represented by 50 reads should be reproducible in technical replicates. To avoid reporting large fold changes due to random variation of counts from low abundance mRNA, RPKM values equivalent to a count of $\leq$ 10 reads per gene were replaced with the average RPKM value equivalent to 10 reads/gene across all the samples in the experiment.

An unpaired two-sample heteroscedastic T-test was performed on the log2 RPKM values to compare the overall effects of Age (PND2 or 4 months) on gene expression. Fold changes were also calculated for 4 months / PND2 using the mean of each group being compared. If the mean of both groups considered in the fold change comparison was below RQT, 'NA' is reported. All statistical analysis was performed using R version 3.2.2 statistical computing software. A total of 7,496 genes were determined to have a low FDR-value (FDR < 0.1) for the unpaired T-Test. Full dataset is available through NCBI GeoDatasets, accession code GSE108083, "RNA-seq analysis of aortic heart valves in mice".

2.2.6 RNA-Sequencing Data Analysis

A heatmap was generated from 23,303 differentially expressed genes. Log2 transformed RPKM values were utilized and hierarchical clustering analysis was performed with Cluster 3.0 software [113]. Genes and samples were clustered using centered correlation as the similarity measure and average linkage as the clustering method. A volcano plot was generated utilizing ggplot2 and is plotted as the -Log10(p-value) vs. Log2 Fold Change. The volcano plot highlights the differential gene expression between postnatal day 2 and 4 month aortic valves. A Venn diagram was generated based only on genes with a low T-Test P value (P<0.05), a fold change >2, and RPKM values above the Reliable Quantification Threshold for all biological replicate samples from either group. If at least one of the gene reads from a triplicate set was proven undetectable while all gene reads in the comparative sample set was proven detectable, the gene was considered to be uniquely expressed. If the gene read from both triplicate sample sets had detectable RPKM values about the Detection Threshold, the gene was considered common amongst sample groups. Genes with at least one triplicate below the Detection Threshold in both sample sets are not represented in the Venn diagram.

Functional annotation was performed through the utilization of Database for Annotation, Visualization, and Integrated Discovery (DAVID) version 6.8 [114]. Differentially expressed genes with an FDR <0.05 and fold change >2 were assessed utilizing Gene Ontology (GO) FAT terms, which were employed to filter out broad GO categories based on a measured specificity of each term. Visualization of GO term analysis was performed using the GOPlot R package version 1.0.2 [115]. To reduce the redundancy of GO terms, the reduce_overlap function was used, with the threshold set to 0.75, which removes GO terms that have a gene overlap greater than or equal to the set threshold. Bubble plots were generated for the reduced GO term list using the GoBubble function, the top 15 GO terms from biological processes, cellular component, and molecular function are visualized. Each bubble represents a term, where the size of the bubble correlates to the number of genes within the term, and it is plotted as –log (FDR) vs. z-score. The z-score is a crude measurement, predicting if a term will be upregulated or downregulated, and is calculated by taking the number of upregulated genes and subtracting the number of downregulated genes and then dividing this number by the square root of the number of genes in each pathway. The circle plot was generated using the GoCircle function, and highlights the gene expression changes within each of the selected terms. The circle plot highlights the overall gene expression change by showing increased expression in red and decreased expression in blue. The circle plot also highlights the p-value of the GO term by the height of the inner rectangle, which is also colored by z-score. A chord plot was generated using the GoChord function, and it represents 59 differentially expressed genes and their correlation to the following associated terms: extracellular matrix, cell proliferation, cell cycle, mitotic cell cycle process, defense response, and regulation of immune system processes. The chord plot also highlights the log fold change of each differentially expressed gene that is shown.

2.2.7 qRT-PCR

RNA was extracted from isolated aortic valves from PND2 and 4 month old *C57BL/6J* mice to validate RNA-seq findings. Briefly, Trizol reagent (Invitrogen) was used to extract RNA according to manufacturer's instructions, and cDNA and PCR reactions were performed as previously described by our lab [116]. Primers for genes selected for validation were designed in NCBI Primer-BLAST based on FASTA sequence:

Table 1: qRT-PCR Primers

Gene Name	Forward Primer Sequence (5' to 3')	Reverse Primer Sequence (5' to 3')
Nid2	AGGAGTGAGCATGTTTCGG	AGGGGTATTGCCAGCTTCAC
Mmp3	TGCATGACAGTGCAAGGGAT	ACACCACACCTGGGCTTATG
Marckls1	CCCGTGAACGGAACAGATGA	CCCACCCTCCTTCCGATTTC
Gsn	GGGACGGCCGGTTACTTAAA	CTTCAGGAATTCGGGGTGCT
Filip1l	AGGCTCCACTGCTGGATTTC	GACTTCTCTGACACGGGACG
Myoc	ACGACACTAAAACGGGGACC	TTCTGGCCTTTGCTGGTAGG
Retnla	GGAACTTCTTGCCAATCCAGC	CAGTGGTCCAGTCAACGAGT
Npdc	GCACTCCCGACACTTTTCTC	GGTACCCACTCCGGGAACT
Sfrp4	CCTGGCAACATACCTGAGCA	AGCATCATCCTTGAACGCCA
Mki67	AGAGCTAACTTGCGCTGACT	ACTCCTTCCAAACAGGCAGG
Nrg1	CCATCTCTCGATGGGCTTCC	ATGCAGAGGCAGAGGCTTAC
Nrep	GCATGATGCCCTTTTTCATCCA	TCCTTAGGCACGGGAAGTCT
Acta2	CCTTCGTGACTACTGCCGAG	GAAGGTAGACAGCGAAGCCA
Dlk1	AGAGTACCCCTCTCCTCACC	CGCCGCTGTTATACTGCAAC
Cfd	TACATGGCTTCCGTGCAAGT	GGGTGAGGCACTACACTCTG

Quantitative real-time PCR (qRT-PCR) using a Step One Plus Real Time PCR system (Applied Biosystems) was used to detect changes in gene expression with Sybr Green reagents. Cycle counts for each target gene were normalized to β-actin expression and differences in gene expression were reported as a fold change from 4 months. Statistical analysis was performed in GraphPad Prism 7.0a.

2.3.1 Postnatal Valve Maturation and Adult Maintenance are Associated with Distinct Transcriptional Profiles

As previously described, the valve structures continue to grow and remodel after birth [2]. As shown here by Movat's Pentachrome stain, murine aortic valve structures at PND2 are thick and composed of predominantly proteoglycan (blue), with less extensive collagen and elastin (Fig. 2A). By 4 months of age, the leaflets have elongated and display distinct layers of collagen (fibrosa, yellow), proteoglycan (blue), and elastin (black) (Fig. 2B).

In order to further define molecular profiles associated with the structural changes in postnatal and 4 month old aortic valves, we performed RNA-sequencing on isolated valve samples. Overall, RNA expression for samples consistently clustered by time point, as shown several ways including a Pearson's correlation matrix, principal component analysis (PCA) and hierarchical heatmap. Of the 23,303 detectable genes, 2,489 were upregulated at the 4-month time point and 2,695 were downregulated. More specifically, 3,659 genes were found to be differentially expressed between the two time points and include 1,858 upregulated and 1,801 downregulated transcripts. Of the 3,659 differentially expressed genes, 602 were unique to the PND2 time point and include *Dlk1*, *Hif3a*, *Agtr2* and *S100A9*, while 477 were only expressed at 4 months (*Cfd*, *Rtn1a*, *Clec3a*, *Adipoq*, *etc.*), leaving 2,580 common to both groups (Fig. 2C). Table 2 includes the top 20 mRNAs uniquely expressed at each time point based on RPKM value, which is indicative of mRNA abundance. Additional RT-qPCR analysis of independent cDNA samples validated trends in RNA-seq findings in 10 out of 12 genes (85%) at a significance threshold of $p<0.05$ (Fig. 2D, 4A, 5A, 5D and data not shown).

2.3.2 Transcriptional Analysis Identified Age-Dependent Transcriptional Profiles and Biological Functions

Heatmap hierarchical clustering analysis, where 23,300 differentially expressed genes and samples were clustered using center correlation as the similarity measurement and average linkage as the clustering method, revealed molecular similarities between biological replicates at each time point and distinct differences between PND2 and 4 months (Fig. 3A). Additional volcano plot analysis graphically displays the differential changes of 23,300 individual transcripts based on significance and fold change (Fig. 3B). To determine functions associated with differential gene expression changes at each time point, Gene Ontology (GO) pathway analysis was performed. The bubble plot in Fig. 3C visualizes the biological processes, cellular components, and molecular functions enriched by the differential data set and the table highlights the top 15 GO terms represented. These include biological processes such as cell proliferation, mitotic cell cycle, and defense response, along with cellular components such as extracellular matrix, indicating that valve maturation involves considerable changes in cell proliferation, ECM composition, and immune system programs. This is further highlighted in Fig. 3D, a circle plot displaying genes which are known to be expressed in the heart valves based on previous publications, and their association with each GO term. More specific trends in these GO terms are shown in Fig. 3E, with individually upregulated and downregulated genes in each category shown as red and blue dots, respectively. The inner rectangles are sized to positively correlate with

29

the significance of each GO term, and colored to represent the overall direction of change in expression of each individual term. For example, the term 'mitotic cell cycle process' has an overall down regulation at 4 months of age, while the 'defense response' has an overall upregulation. In contrast, the 'extracellular matrix' GO term is overall neither up-, nor downregulated, but the change in many individual transcripts is significant. Together these genomic analyses have defined transcriptional profiles of PND2 and 4-month aortic valve structures and identified changes in functions associated with these mRNA patterns.

2.3.3 Proliferation Programs are Downregulated in 4 Month Old Aortic Valves

Based on enrichment of cell proliferation-related genes from GO analysis (Table 3), we first validated the fold change trends observed by RNA-seq using RT-qPCR (Fig. 4A) on independent biological samples. These validated genes include three positive regulators of proliferation *mKi67, Nrg1* and *Marckls*, which all decreased in 4 month old aortic valves, and an anti-proliferative gene, *Sfrp4*, found to have increased expression at this time point (Fig. 4A) [117-120]. To further validate mRNA findings, we utilized 5-ethynyl-2'-deoxyuridine (EdU) to visualize and compare the number of cells actively undergoing mitosis in the aortic valve at PND2 and 4 months of age (Fig. 4B). At the earlier time point, ~10.5% of cells were found to be EdU-positive, while only 0.16% of cells were proliferating at 4 months (Fig. 4B-D). These data are consistent with transcriptional changes and previous reports from our lab [60]. Together, these observations suggest that a decline in cell division at 4 months is due to a combination of decreasing expression of postnatal proliferation programs while simultaneously increasing adult programs which inhibit proliferation.

*2.3.4 Postnatal and Adult Aortic Valves Have Distinct Extracellular Matrix mRNA
Programs*

As indicated by the GO term z-score in Fig. 3C and 3E, the overall expression of
ECM transcripts does not significantly increase or decrease with age, yet there are
considerable differences in the specific ECM-related mRNAs that are expressed between
the two time points (Table 4). Matrix metalloproteinases, or Mmps, are known to be
expressed in both healthy and diseased valves and are associated with physiological and
pathological remodeling of the ECM respectively [121-123]. Also known as stromelysin-
1, Mmp3 targets degradation of proteoglycans, collagens, and elastins [124] and this Mmp
family member has been described in cancer [125, 126], but little is known about Mmp3
in mouse valves. In this study, *Mmp3* increased from 1.22 reads per million kilobases
(RPKM) at PND2 to 86.14 RPKM at 4 months. This significant increase was confirmed
by RT-qPCR (Fig. 5A) and immunofluorescence of AoV tissue sections, where it is
localized primarily to the sub-endothelial region of the leaflet (Fig. 5B). Conversely, the
basement membrane ECM protein *Nidogen 2* (*Nid2*) was more highly detected in PND2
samples at 76 RPKM, while only 15 RPKM were detected at 4 months. This expression
pattern was confirmed by RT-qPCR (Fig. 5D) and immunofluorescence data, which shows
broad Nid2 localization towards the ventricularis edge at PND2, but within the fibrosa layer
region at 4 months (Fig. 5E, F). These data show that PND2 and 4 month old aortic valves
have distinct ECM-related transcriptional profiles associated with growth and maintenance
respectively.

2.3.5 Gene Ontology Defense Response Markers are Highly Enriched in 4 Month Old Aortic Valves

As shown in Fig. 6A and Table 5, a large majority (77%) of defense response genes are most highly expressed in aortic valve structures at 4 months of age and include *Ccl19*, *Ptgs2* and *Cxcl9*. The increased expression of *Ptgs2* (also known as *Cox2*) (Fig. 6B, C) and *Rarres2* (also known as *Tig2*) (Fig. 6D, E) are confirmed here by immunofluorescence. Ptgs2 is an enzyme involved in the synthesis of prostaglandins which are known to mediate pain and inflammation responses [127], and has been described in the valve as a pro-osteogenic marker [128]. Consistent with this previous valve study, we observed expression in the endothelium at 4 months of age (Fig. 6C). Like Ptgs2, Rarres2 is also known to regulate inflammation and has been linked with hypertension [129], a known risk factor of aortic valve stenosis [130]. By immunofluorescence, Rarres2 is widely expressed throughout the valve leaflet at 4 months of age. Overall, our RNA-seq data shows that expression of defense response-related genes increases with age in the murine aortic valve.

2.4 Discussion

This current study explores transcriptional differences in PND2 and 4 month old murine aortic valve expression profiles with the goal of identifying genetic programs representative of valve growth and valve maintenance, respectively. Long term, this may be important for the development of alternative therapies; specifically, those exploring the growth or regenerative capacity of adult, diseased valves. Our results indicate that at PND2, dynamic leaflet growth is associated with a unique transcriptional profile compared to homeostatic adult valves at 4 months. Of the 23,303 detectable genes in our RNA-seq data, the number of differentially expressed transcripts found to be up and down regulated at each time point were approximately equal, suggesting that gene transcription patterns were not overtly altered, but rather transitioned from a postnatal to adult expression profile. Such profiles are related to enriched biological functions including cell proliferation at PND2 and defense response at 4 months of age. Interestingly, ECM components were enriched at both time points, but the associated mRNA profiles were unique. Together these analyses provide critical information related to genetic programs in the growing and homeostatic heart valve.

Previous analyses have shown that compared to adult stages, the postnatal heart valve is characterized by high levels of cell proliferation, as well as efficient VEC function as indicated by nitric oxide bioavailability, low permeability, and intact mitochondria [60]. Here, we contribute to this current knowledge and further advance our understanding of the molecular signatures and biological functions characteristic of the whole aortic valve structure at PND2 and 4 months.

PND2 murine aortic valves are defined by a specific transcriptional profile including the unique expression of 602 genes (Fig. 2C, Table 2) that were not detected at 4 months of age. In addition, 1,801 transcripts were upregulated at PND2, while 1,858 were decreased compared to the adult homeostatic valve. According to GO analysis, many of the transcripts enriched at PND2 suggest an overall enrichment of active cell proliferation by a specific set of genes. These include those associated with active cell division (*Ki67*) as well as pro-proliferation markers including *Bub1* and *Cdk1* [131], *Foxm1*, [132], and *Nrg1*, [118] and inhibitors *Nox4* [133, 134], and *Sfrp4* [135, 136]. This specific expression profile of cell proliferation markers supports EdU observations and represents active elongation of the immature valve structure. It will become important to understand how this gene profile is regulated following PND2 to avoid hyperplasia of the valve structures and disruption of structure-function relationships. To our knowledge, this is the first study to define the molecular signature of cell proliferation in postnatal valves and this may be important for examining potential mechanisms to stimulate cell proliferation in the adult to replenish or replace healthy cell populations in damaged or dysfunctional valves.

In addition to high levels of cell proliferation, the PND2 valve is characterized by a specific ECM mRNA profile (Table 4) which likely corresponds the mechanical demands during the postnatal period. Pentachrome staining (Fig. 2A) shows the classic overview of the postnatal valve structure predominately composed of proteoglycans as indicated by extensive alcian blue staining and confirmed by high transcriptional levels of the proteoglycans aggrecan (*ACAN)* and versican (*VCAN*). When comparing PND2 to 4 months, RNA-seq analysis reveals significant enrichment of highly expressed fibrillar collagens including *Col24a1*, *Col9a1*, and *Col5a1* at PND2, indicating the need for additional stability as the growing postnatal valve adapts to hemodynamic changes in response to closing of the foramen ovale [137, 138]. RNA-seq analysis also uncovered higher PND2 levels of ECM proteins such as *Frem1/Frem2* and nidogen2 (*Nid2*), which have been shown to stabilize basement membranes underlying endothelial cells and may provide further structural integrity to the developing valve [139, 140]. Interestingly, we see higher elastin (*Eln*) mRNA levels at PND2 than at 4 months, although this is not reflected in Pentachrome staining (Fig. 2A), suggesting that elastin transcription occurs in advance of protein deposition and organization in the valve structure. Besides identifying the enrichment of differentially expressed fibrillary collagens and specific proteoglycans, PND2 valve also expresses a distinct profile of ECM enzymes, such as *Mmp15* and *Adamts17*, indicating the need for physiological remodeling during growth and maturation. An important consideration for future work will involve the integral relationship between VIC age and phenotype and ECM composition of the valve. Together, our data has begun to elucidate connections between postnatal physiological cues, VIC proliferation, and ECM profile.

The 4 month adult valve is physically and molecularly distinct from the postnatal valve, with elongated leaflets containing distinct layers of collagen, proteoglycan, and elastin (Fig. 2B). At this time point, 477 transcripts were found to be uniquely expressed, with the most abundant unique mRNAs including *Cfd*, *Retnla*, and *Clec3a*. In contrast to the PND2 aortic valve, the adult valve displays significantly decreased levels of cell proliferation. This is likely due to increased expression of proliferation inhibitors including *Nox4* and *Sfrp,4* and lack of enrichment of positive regulators of proliferation. However, there is some degree of cell division as detected by EdU analysis showing ~0.16%, and these levels are comparable to proliferation rates of other adult cardiac tissues [141]. Together this switch in the cell proliferation is likely important for maintaining homeostasis of established valve cell populations and the physiological response to normal wear-and-tear [142].

At 4 months of age, the valve ECM is diverse compared to PND2 (Table 4) and likely reflects differences in biomechanical demand in response to the adult circulatory system [143, 144]. Similar to the PND2 valve, collagens and proteoglycans are predominant, however at 4 months, the most highly, differentially expresses collagens are those associated with basement membranes (and not fibrillary) including *Col4a6* and *Col18a1*, which act as a cell scaffold to maintain current cell populations and cell integrity as opposed to providing support for high cell turnover. In addition, the proteoglycan profile is moved towards enrichment of decorin (*Dcn*) and biglycan (*Bgn*) consistent with previous studies in aging pigs [145]. Furthermore, the cocktail of ECM remodeling enzymes is shifted to *Mmp3* and its inhibitor *Timp3* at 4 months, possibly indicating a differential need of the ECM to sustain homeostasis. Previous studies have suggested correlations between VIC phenotype and ECM composition [57, 66] and therefore we anticipate that our findings at 4 months are related to the quiescent VICs, while the diversity at PND2 is dictated by proliferative and active VICs.

One of the most prominent differences in expression profiles between the PND2 and 4 month AoV is the considerable upregulation of defense-related transcripts at the older time point, indicating increased immune system activation with valve maturation (Fig. 6, Table 5). Previous studies from other groups have shown that the appearance of immune markers such as *Ptgs2* and *Rarres2* precedes the onset of disease both in the heart valve and other cardiovascular systems [128, 129]. In addition, there is increasing evidence to suggest that inflammation in the valve is an initial homeostatic repair mechanism activated in response to minor valve injuries sustained throughout life, but that this repair mechanism may become pathogenic if overactive or long-lasting (reviewed [146]). Our study suggests that some level of activation of the immune system in the valve is present at 4 months of age under homeostatic conditions, however, it is not clear whether these defense markers are an early indication of valve degeneration, or a root cause of disease themselves. Further investigation into target genes such as *Cfd* and *Adipoq* will give insight into the possible role of defense response genes in valve disease therapeutics.

Valve disease is complex and likely has many underlying causes. However, one commonality is the dysfunction or loss of healthy valve cells, which results in an inability to maintain structure-function relationships. Therefore, the ability to replenish healthy valve cell populations would be a distinct therapeutic advantage. Our data shows that postnatal heart valves contain highly proliferative VICs producing a distinctive set of postnatal ECM proteins, while adult VICs are mainly quiescent and are associated with a very different ECM composition as well as increased defense response markers. This presents multiple conceivable methods for promoting healthy valve cell replenishment during disease: upregulation of postnatal proliferation programs, promoting formation of appropriate ECM, or downregulation of adult immune programs. Further research needs to be done to elucidate specific regulators in each of these categories and to determine complimentary therapeutic approaches.

Table 2: Top 20 Unique Genes at PND2 and 4 Month Time Points
Genes are listed in order of RPKM with the most highly expressed at the top of the list.

PND2	4 Month
Dlk1	Cfd
Hif3a	2210407C18Rik
Agtr2	Retnla
S100a9	Clec3a
Slc38a5	Adipoq
Col24a1	Ces1d
Bmp7	Thrsp
Vash2	Pck1
Igf2bp3	Mgl2
Stfa1	C7
S100a8	Inmt
Cited1	Cidec
Gm5483	Fmo3
Frem2	Angpt4
Gipr	Hamp
Ube2c	Art1
Dctd	Tmem45b
1110032F04Rik	Olfr224
C1qtnf3	Plin1
Cdkn3	Rpl31

Table 3: Top 20 Genes Included in the "Cell Proliferation" GO Term
Genes are sorted according to fold change, with the highest fold change at the top of the list.

Downregulated at 4mo	Upregulated at 4 mo
AGTR2	ADIPOQ
H19	HSPA1A
BMP7	CD74
VASH2	PLA2G2D
IGF2	RBP4
IGF2BP1	H2-AA
FAM83D	H2-AB1
CTHRC1	VSIG4
CRH	CCL19
CDK1	CRLF1
NRK	CCL11
BEX1	NOX4
BUB1	SFRP4
IL31RA	CD209A
MELK	PTGFR
SCUBE2	BCL6
CCNB1	ITGAX
FIGNL1	KCNA1
AURKB	LGI4
UHRF1	ATF3

Table 4: Top 20 Genes Included in the "Extracellular Matrix" GO Term
Genes are sorted according to fold change, with the highest fold change at the top of the list.

Downregulated at 4mo	Upregulated at 4 mo
S100A9	MYOC
COL24A1	MMP3
BMP7	GLDN
2010005H15RIK	CHAD
CTHRC1	MMP10
FREM2	COMP
COL26A1	ENTPD2
ELN	LAMC3
COL9A1	CILP2
FREM1	SOD3
ADAMTS12	FBLN7
FRAS1	NPNT
MFAP2	PRELP
ADAMTS17	MMP12
WISP1	COL4A6
HMCN1	VIT
LAMA1	CCBE1
COL12A1	CPXM2
ACAN	OPTC
TNC	SERPINF1

Table 5: Top 20 Genes Included in the "Defense Response" GO Term
Genes are sorted according to fold change, with the highest fold change at the top of the list.

Downregulated at 4mo	Upregulated at 4mo
AGTR2	CFD
S100A9	ADIPOQ
CITED1	HAMP
IGF2	HP
COLEC10	CD74
NGP	CCL8
C1QTNF3	H2-AA
CRH	H2-EB1
S100A8	H2-AB1
IL31RA	CLEC10A
ADAMTS12	GM2564
CHAF1B	CCL19
AGER	CCL11
PBK	C4B
ULBP1	C4A
RNASEL	PTGFR
RAET1E	BCL6
ELF3	ITGAX
BRINP1	PTGS2
RAET1D	ESR1

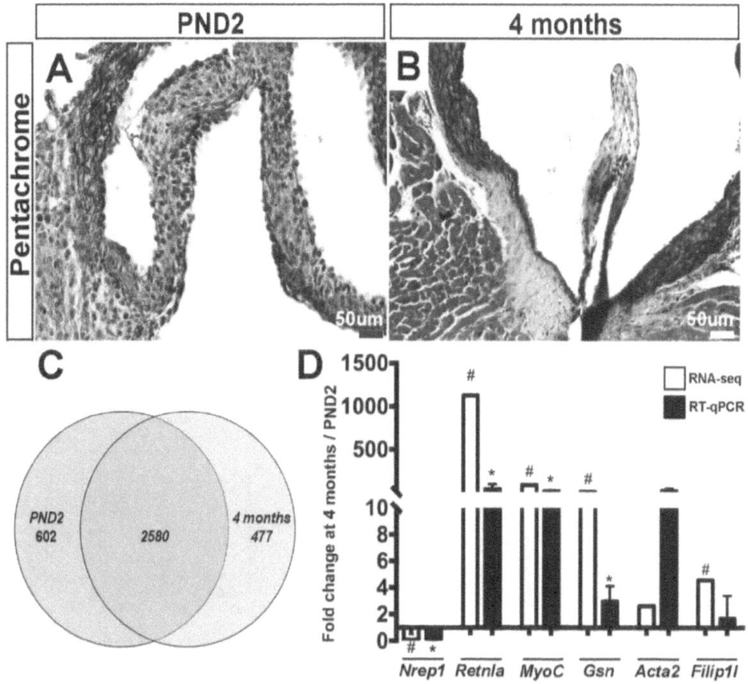

Figure 2: Postnatal and Adult Aortic Valves Display Differences in ECM Composition and Gene Expression.

Movat's Pentachrome staining to show ECM composition at PND2 **(A)** and 4 months **(B)** (black: elastic fibers and cell nuclei, blue: proteoglycans, yellow: collagen, red: muscle and fibrinoids). **(C)** Venn diagram to show distribution of the detected mRNAs that were uniquely, or commonly expressed at PND2 or 4 months. **(D)** RT-qPCR validation (black bars) of RNA-seq findings (white bars) (n=3, *:p<0.05; two-tailed unpaired t-test, #:FDR<0.05).

42

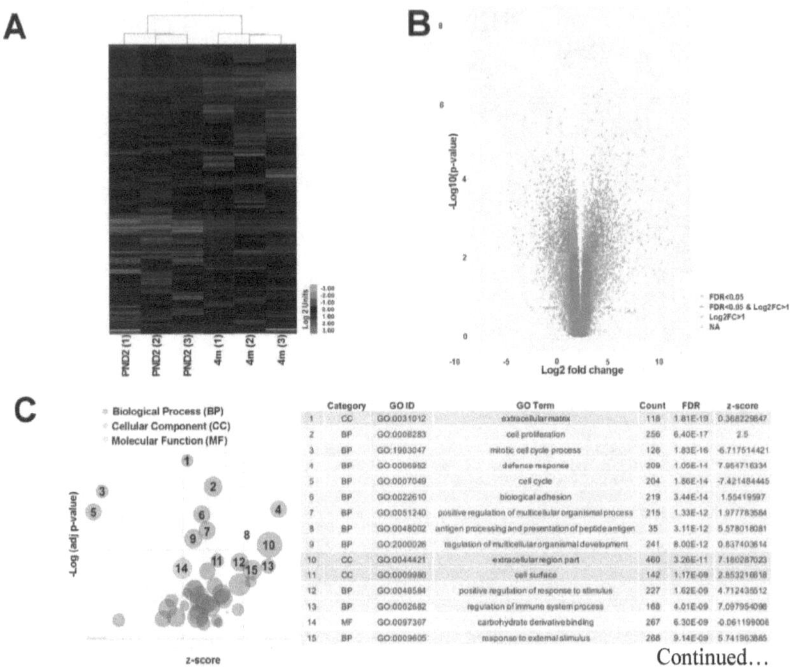

	Category	GO ID	GO Term	Count	FDR	z-score
1	CC	GO:0031012	extracellular matrix	118	1.81E-19	0.368229847
2	BP	GO:0008283	cell proliferation	256	6.40E-17	2.5
3	BP	GO:1903047	mitotic cell cycle process	126	1.83E-16	-6.717514421
4	BP	GO:0006952	defense response	209	1.05E-14	7.964716334
5	BP	GO:0007049	cell cycle	204	1.86E-14	-7.421484445
6	BP	GO:0022610	biological adhesion	219	3.44E-14	1.55419597
7	BP	GO:0051240	positive regulation of multicellular organismal process	215	1.33E-12	1.977783584
8	BP	GO:0048002	antigen processing and presentation of peptide antigen	35	3.11E-12	5.578018081
9	BP	GO:2000026	regulation of multicellular organismal development	241	8.00E-12	0.837403614
10	CC	GO:0044421	extracellular region part	460	3.26E-11	7.180287023
11	CC	GO:0009986	cell surface	142	1.17E-09	2.853216618
12	BP	GO:0048584	positive regulation of response to stimulus	227	1.62E-09	4.712435512
13	BP	GO:0002682	regulation of immune system process	168	4.01E-09	7.097954098
14	MF	GO:0097367	carbohydrate derivative binding	267	6.30E-09	-0.061199008
15	BP	GO:0009605	response to external stimulus	288	9.14E-09	5.741963885

Continued…

Figure 3: RNA-Seq Analysis Reveals Transcriptomic Differences Between PND2 and 4 Month Old Murine Aortic Valves.

(A) Hierarchical heatmap cluster to show clustering of biological replicates (n=3). (B) Volcano plot of differentially regulated genes sorted according to fold change and significance (FDR). Green dots represent genes with log2 fold change >1 and FDR<0.05. (C) Gene ontology (GO) analysis reveals top differentially regulated GO terms, displayed according to significance (p-value) and z-score, a measure of overall up or down regulation for the category. Data represented as a bubble plot (left). The size of each circle represents the number of differentially expressed genes, while color represents the category. Table (right) lists the top GO terms along with count, FDR, and z-score. (D) Chord plot showing 59 differentially expressed genes previously associated with healthy and diseased valves, and their overlap between significant GO terms as determined in (C). (E) Circular plot highlighting gene expression differences within each selected GO term, with each red dot depicting a gene upregulated at 4 months in that category, and each blue dot showing a gene downregulated at 4 months. The height of the inner rectangle represents the p-value of the GO term and is colored according to z-score.

43

Continued…

D
extracellular
matrix
cell
proliferation
cell
cycle
mitotic cell
cycle process
defense
response
regulation of immune
system process
Log Fold Change
E
regulation of
immune system
process
extracellular
matrix
cell
surface
cell
proliferation
biological
adhesion
mitotic cell
cycle process
cell
cycle
defense
response
z-score
-7.42
7.95
logFC
downregulated
upregulated

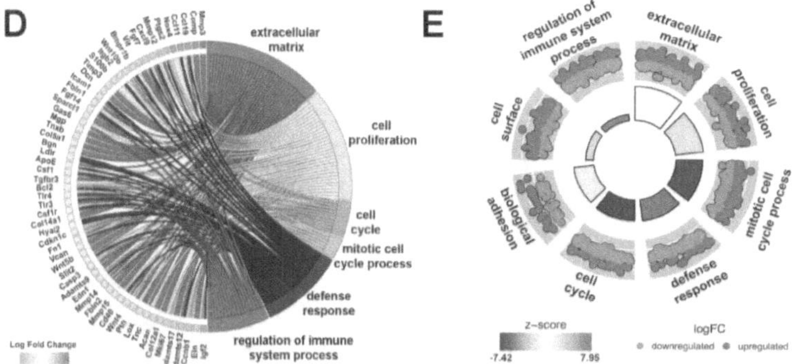

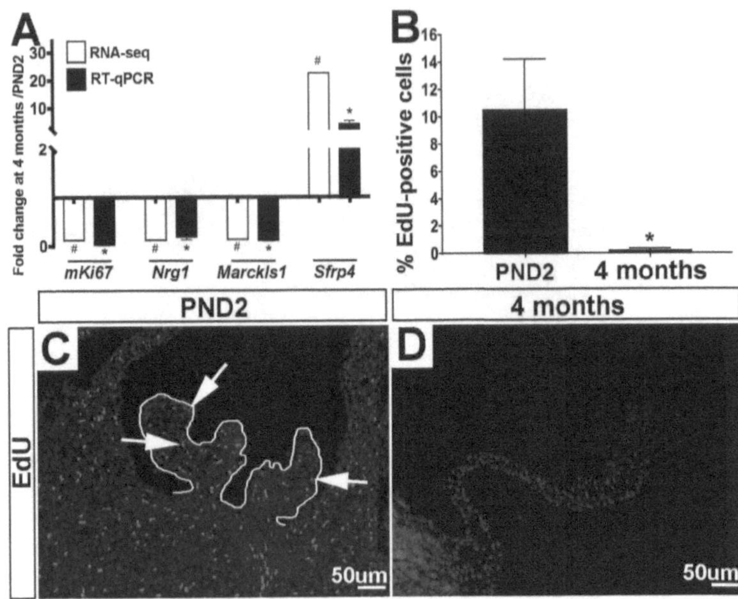

Figure 4: Positive Regulators of Cell Proliferation are Enriched in PND2 Murine Aortic Heart Valves.

(A) RT-qPCR performed on independent samples (black bars) validates the RNA-seq fold change (white bars) trends for proliferation-related genes. Expression is normalized to 1, indicated by the x-axis. (n=3, *:p<0.05; two-tailed unpaired t-test, #:FDR<0.05). (B) Quantification of EdU-positive cells as a percentage of total cell nuclei (indicated by DAPI, blue) at PND2 and 4 month time points. (n=3, *:p<0.05, two-tailed unpaired t-test). (C) Representative images of staining for incorporation of EdU into replicating DNA (white arrows point to EdU-positive cells) reveals high levels of proliferation in PND2 AoV as compared to (D) EdU staining in 4 month AoV.

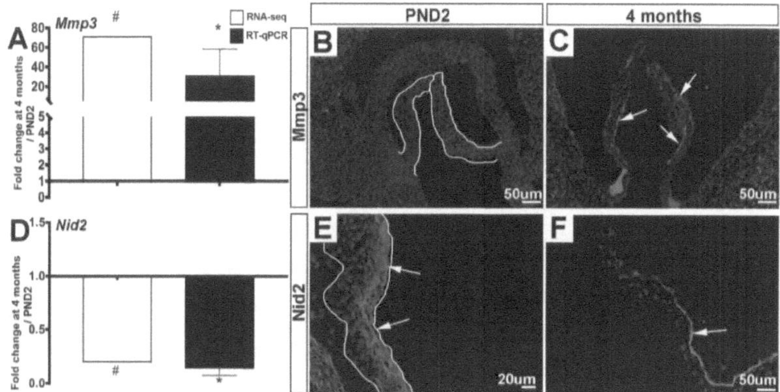

Figure 5: ECM Molecular Profiles Between PND2 and 4 Month Old Murine Aortic Valves are Distinct.

(A) RT-qPCR performed on independent samples (black bars) validates the trends seen in RNA-seq data (white bars). Expression is normalized to 1, indicated by the x-axis (n=3, *:p<0.05; two-tailed unpaired t-test, #:FDR<0.05). **(B)** Immunofluorescence staining for Mmp3 reveals low expression at PND2 compared to **(C)** 4 months (white arrows indicate Mmp3-positive cells). **(D)** RT-qPCR performed on independent samples (black bars) validates the trends seen in RNA-seq data (white bars) for ECM gene *Nid2*. Expression is normalized to 1, indicated by the x-axis (n=3, *:p<0.05; two-tailed unpaired t-test, #:FDR<0.05). **(E)** Immunofluorescence staining for Nid2 reveals high expression at PND2 (white arrows indicate Nid2-positive cells) compared to **(F)** Nid2 staining at the 4-month time point.

46

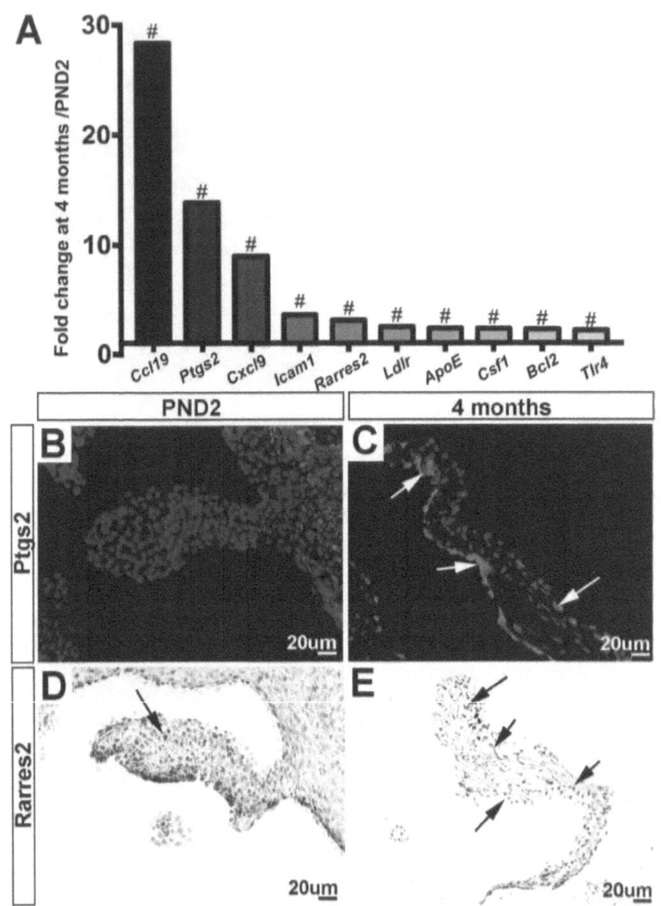

Figure 6: Expression of Defense-Related Genes Increases with Valve Maturation
(**A**) RNA-sequencing fold changes of defense-related genes. Expression is normalized to 1, indicated by the x-axis (#:FDR<0.05). (**B**) Immunofluorescence staining for Ptgs2 validates RNA-seq trends, showing low expression at PND2 compared to (**C**) Ptgs2 staining at the 4-month time point (white arrows indicate Ptgs2-positive cells). (**D**) Immunofluorescence staining for Rarres2 validates RNA-seq trends, showing low expression at PND2 compared to (**E**) Rarres2 staining at the 4 month time point.

Chapter 3: Exploring the Reparative Response of the Injured Heart Valve Endothelium

3.1 Introduction

The aortic valve (AoV) consists of three cusps composed of highly organized layers of extracellular matrix (ECM) containing collagens, proteoglycans, and elastin. Together, this arrangement provides the biomechanical functions necessary for efficient opening and closing during the cardiac cycle [2, 3, 9]. Maintenance of the composition and organization of the ECM layers is critical for ensuring proper valve structure and function throughout life, and pathological disturbances underlie structural and biomechanical failure of the cusps, which left untreated can lead to heart failure or even death. [3, 14, 147].

Production and maintenance of the valve ECM is mediated by a population of fibroblast-like valve interstitial cells (VICs) which reside within the interior of the valve cusp. VICs are a heterogenous population with multiple embryonic origins including endothelial, myocardial, and neural crest lineages [15, 16]. In the absence of disease, this cell population is quiescent and functions to maintain turnover of the valve ECM in response to normal wear-and-tear [58, 59] through a balance of degradation and synthesis [18]. However, activation of the VIC population has been reported during normal embryonic valve development but also abnormally in disease. The function of an activated VIC is not clear, but previous studies suggest a role in active remodeling of the ECM [6, 17, 57]. During embryonic development, this process is well-balanced and results in establishment of the essential stratified ECM layers [2]. However, disease-related remodeling is likely pathological and can lead to severe disruption of the ECM structure and functional impairment [3, 148]. In addition to the VIC population, approximately 10% of cells within the valve interstitium are CD45-positive immune cells [36]. These bone marrow-derived cells do not appear to have an inflammatory function and their role is likely involved in the maintenance of the adult valve in the absence of disease [34, 36, 149]. Overall, the phenotypes of the cells within the valve cusp require precise regulation in order to preserve structure-function relationships throughout life.

In addition to the interstitium, each valve cusp is surrounded by a single layer of valve endothelial cells (VECs) which play a crucial role in adult valve maintenance and disease prevention [22, 23, 72]. This impermeable endothelial layer restricts infiltration of inflammatory cells and circulating risk factors which are thought to trigger pathogenic processes within the valve [14, 22, 23]. In addition, the VECs serve as a signaling source and produce secretory growth factors and other signaling molecules received by underlying VICs to maintain their quiescence and regulate downstream target genes involved in ECM homeostasis [24-26, 32]. As function of the endothelium is essential for normal valve maintenance, any disruption or impairment of the endothelial layer is detrimental and promotes pathological changes in VIC phenotypes which lead to ECM alterations. Histological studies of human valves isolated at end-stage disease have demonstrated a link between the severity of biomechanical failure and the level of endothelial disruption [75, 150]. Additionally, work from our group has shown that as mice age, the morphology of the AoV endothelial layer becomes compromised and the VECs begin to exhibit dysfunctional phenotypes. This study established a connection between VEC dysfunction and the increased frequency of valve disease in the elderly [60]. Further examinations have moved beyond analyzing associations and have established endothelial disruption as an underlying cause of valve disease. Investigations in mice conclude that direct genetic manipulation of VECs promotes the onset of ECM remodeling and functional deterioration of the valve [26, 58]. Additionally, severe mechanical damage to the valve endothelium has served as a model for accelerated AoV disease in otherwise healthy mice [76], and surgical procedures such as balloon valvuloplasty have also been shown to injure the human valve endothelium and result in abnormal ECM changes within the valve cusps [151, 152]. Together, this data indicates that both molecular dysfunction and physical disruption of the valve endothelium can contribute to disease development. Overall, these collective studies suggest that VEC impairment plays a significant role in the onset and progression of valve disease.

The standard treatment for end-stage valve disease continues to be surgical repair or replacement. Although there have been attempts at the use of non-surgical treatments such as statin therapy, these trials have not shown a consistent positive impact on valve function [81-84]. As surgery can include risks and disadvantages, the search for effective non-surgical treatments remains a priority. As described above, the requirement for a healthy endothelial layer to promote proper valve homeostasis suggests that repair of the damaged VEC layer could represent a promising path towards development of pharmaceutical valve disease therapies. Studies in the analogous vascular endothelial system have shown relatively robust repair capacity after endothelial injury and have elucidated pathways and mechanisms which may soon be therapeutically targeted [98, 153]. Comparatively, the field of valvular endothelial injury and repair is still in early stages and few studies exist in the literature. Two recent publications from the Stainier [100] and Beis [99] groups focus on regeneration of the zebrafish atrioventricular valve after genetically-induced VIC ablation, but do not emphasize damage or repair of the VEC layer in these animals, which are known for having considerable regenerative capacity. Earlier publications also confirm the ability of untreated valve cells in *ex vivo* culture to physically repair the endothelial layer within 2 days of a denudation injury on the surface of the valve [101, 154]. Based on the current state of the field and our understanding of valvular biology, it appears that activation of endogenous endothelial repair programs may provide a promising route for *in vivo* non-surgical therapeutic treatment for valve disease. However, more work is required to fully understand the process of valve endothelial injury and repair, particularly in models comparable to humans which are traditionally considered non-regenerative, such as adult mice.

To address these gaps in the field, we adapted a murine surgical model of mechanical valve endothelial injury [76] to produce mild damage in order to examine the response of the AoV and investigate the potential for self-repair and prevention of disease. With this model, we demonstrate a robust short-term injury response following mild damage to the endothelium in adult wild type mice and examine the associated transcriptional changes and biological processes. Using a genetic mouse model, we confirm the involvement of a key signaling protein, Cthrc1, which we identified as part of the signaling response mechanism. Additionally, we investigate the injury response in aging mice to better understand how existing endothelial dysfunction affects the ability to repair. Overall, this study is one of the first to explore the potential for valve self-repair following injury and to elucidate the mechanisms underlying this potential beneficial response in a mammalian model.

3.2 Materials and Methods

3.2.1 Mice

Adult (2-4 months old) and aging adult (16-18 months old) *C57BL/6J* mice were purchased from Jackson Laboratories (#0064). Adult (2-4 months old) *Cthrc1$^{-/-}$* mice were obtained by breeding *Cthrc1$^{+/-}$* mice which were a generous gift from Dr. Volkhard Linder at the Maine Medical Center Research Institute. Mice were fed regular chow mix and housed in a controlled environment with 12-hour light/dark cycles at 21°C and 23% humidity and water ad libitum. Animals were euthanized by CO_2 exposure followed by secondary euthanasia by cervical dislocation (adult mice). All animal procedures were approved by The Research Institute at Nationwide Children's Hospital (NCH) and Medical College of Wisconsin (MCW) Institutional Animal Care and Use Committees (Protocol # AR13-00054 (NCH) and AUA00006769 (MCW)).

3.2.2 Endothelial Wire Injury

This procedure was adapted from Honda et al. [76]. Anesthesia was induced in mice with 3% isoflurane with 1 liter per minute oxygen and maintained throughout the surgery with 2% isoflurane at 1 liter per minute oxygen. Mice received a dose of buprenorphine consistent with body weight (0.03mg/kg for standard buprenorphine or 1.5mg/kg for sustained release (SR) buprenorphine). Hair was removed from the mouse chest with a chemical hair remover. After sterilization of the surgery site, a small incision (<2cm) was made in the neck region of the mouse and the right carotid artery isolated by blunt dissection. A thin 0.36mm angioplasty wire (Asahi Intecc #AG14M345) was introduced into the right carotid artery and advanced into the aorta and through the AoV into the left ventricle (LV). The wire was then visualized by echocardiography in the parasternal long axis (PLAX) view (see below). To induce mild AoV injury, the wire was moved in and out of the AoV opening in a "scratching" motion 20 times, then re-inserted through the valve opening into the LV and rotated 20 times for a "spinning" motion. The wire was then carefully removed, and the right carotid artery ligated with 5-0 braided silk sutures (Ethicon #A302H) to prevent blood loss. The incision was then sutured closed using 4-0 coated VICRYL sutures (Ethicon #VCP422H) and the mouse removed from anesthesia and allowed to recover with heat assistance before returning to the animal care facility. The sham surgery consisted of the same procedure with the wire only advanced to the aorta and not across the AoV opening.

3.2.3 In Vivo *Echocardiography*

General

Baseline echocardiography was performed in all animals no more than 1 week before the wire injury procedure, and serial echocardiography was performed in animals at either 5 hours post-injury (hpi), or at 24hpi, 72hpi, 1 week post-injury, 2 weeks post-injury and 4 weeks post-injury. Anesthesia was induced in mice with 3% isoflurane with 1 liter per minute oxygen, and maintained with 2% isoflurane with 1 liter per minute oxygen. Anesthetized mice were secured to a heating platform in the supine position and chest hair was removed via chemical hair remover. A warm echocardiography gel was placed on the chest wall to enhance sound transduction, and a small echocardiographic sound wave transducer was placed on the anterior chest wall. Electrocardiogram (ECG) electrodes were placed in a standard limb configuration to monitor heart rate. Body temperature was monitored by the use of a rectal probe and controlled with a heat lamp and heating platform described above. Ultrasound images were obtained using a Visual Sonics Vevo 2100 imaging system at 30 MHz or a Visual Sonics Vevo 3100 imaging system at 30 MHz.

Wire Injury Procedure

To aid insertion of the guidewire through the AoV opening during the wire injury procedure, the AoV was visualized in the PLAX view. View of the wire, LV, and AoV were maintained throughout the procedure beginning when the wire was inserted until the wire was removed, approximately 5 minutes.

Functional Measurements

Heart rate, cardiac output, left ventricular end systolic volume, left ventricular end diastolic volume, left ventricular end systolic diameter, and left ventricular end diastolic diameter were determined from M-mode short axis views at the level of the papillary muscles. Aortic diameter was measured by M-mode in a PLAX view of the ascending aorta. E/A ratios were captured by pulse wave Doppler on flow over the mitral valve. AoV velocity was captured from a suprasternal notch view in a right high parasternal location for optimal interrogation of the AoV. Aortic regurgitation was assessed via color and flow Doppler and was only considered positive if present in both modes. The entire echocardiography procedure lasted approximately 10-15 minutes, after which mice recovered from anesthesia with heat assistance and were returned to the animal care facility. If the echocardiogram occurred on the day of a sacrifice, mice were allowed to recover prior to tissue harvest. Echocardiography statistics were measured by 2-way ANOVA with multiple comparisons.

3.2.4 Evans Blue Dye AoV Permeability

Evans Blue Dye (EBD) was utilized to assess permeability of the AoV endothelial barrier. For the 6-hour post-surgery timepoint, EBD was injected immediately after surgery via retro-orbital injection and hearts were harvested 6 hours later. For the 48 hour and 4 week post-surgery timepoints, EBD was injected 24 hours before sacrifice via tail vein injection. For all timepoints, $100\mu l$ of a $0.2\mu m$ filtered 1% w/v solution of EBD (Sigma-Aldrich #E2129) in sterile saline was injected. EBD fluorescence on frozen tissue sections was visualized with an EVOS M7000 microscope and quantified (see below).

3.2.5 Immunohistochemistry and Immunofluorescence
Antibody Immunofluorescence

For histology experiments unless otherwise stated, hearts were collected from young and aging mice at relevant timepoints and immediately embedded and frozen in OCT medium (Sakura Finetek #4583), then sectioned at $7\mu m$. Sections containing the AoV were then subjected to EBD visualization (see above) or immunofluorescence staining. For cryosections, slides were fixed in 4% paraformaldehyde/1xPBS for 20 minutes at room temperature and subsequently permeabilized using 0.1% triton-X 100 (Sigma-Aldrich T9284) in 1xPBS. Sections were then subjected to blocking for 1 hour at room temperature in blocking solution (1% BSA, 1% cold water fish skin gelatin, 0.1% Tween-20/PBS) and incubated overnight at 4°C or 1 hour at room temperature with indicated primary antibodies diluted in a 1:1 solution of 1xPBS and blocking solution (Table 6). For Cthrc1 and Tgfβ1 immunofluorescence, antibodies required the use of formalin fixed, paraffin embedded (FFPE) tissue. For FFPE processing, hearts were collected from young and aging mice 48 hours post-injury and fixed in 4% paraformaldehyde/1xPBS overnight at 4°C, then embedded in paraffin wax and sectioned at 7μm. Paraffin was removed in xylenes, and tissue sections were rehydrated through a graded ethanol series and rinsed in 1xPBS. Sections containing the AoV were then subjected to antigen retrieval by boiling for 10 minutes in unmasking solution (Vector Laboratories #H-3300), blocking for 1 hour at room temperature as described above, and incubated overnight at 4°C with indicated antibodies diluted in a 1:1 solution of 1xPBS and blocking solution (Table 6).

Table 6: Antibodies Used for Tissue Immunofluorescence

Antibody (α)	Raised In	Company, Product #	Dilution	Section Type
Versican V0, V1	Rabbit	Invitrogen #PA1-1748A	1:200	Cryo
Phospho-histone H3	Rabbit	Sigma-Aldrich #06-570	1:200	Cryo
VE-cadherin	Goat	R&D Systems #AF1002	1:100	Cryo
CD45	Goat	R&D Systems #AF114	1:100	Cryo
Cthrc1	Rabbit	MMCRI #Vli55	1:100	FFPE
Tgfβ1	Rabbit	Novus Biologicals #NBP1-80289	1:100	FFPE

For primary antibody detection, sections were incubated for 1 hour at room temperature with appropriate secondary antibodies including Alexa Fluor 488 or Alexa Fluor 568 donkey α rabbit and donkey α goat (1:400, LifeTechnologies), then mounted in

Vectashield anti-fade medium with DAPI (Vector Laboratories #H-1500) to detect cell nuclei.

Collagen Hybridizing Peptide

For collagen hybridizing peptide (CHP) immunofluorescence, cryosections were collected as described above. Sections were then fixed in 4% paraformaldehyde/1xPBS for 20 minutes at room temperature. To detect complete or total collagen, tissue sections were subjected to heat treatment by placing in ddH_2O and boiling for 10 minutes in a microwave. Sections were subsequently permeabilized in 0.1% triton-X 100 (Sigma-Aldrich #T9284) in 1xPBS and then blocked as described above for 1 hours at room temperature. Next, a 15µm dilution of 5-FAM conjugated CHP (Advanced BioMatrix #5264) in 1xPBS was heated for 5 minutes at 80°C and immediately cooled on ice before adding 50µl of solution to each section and incubating overnight at 4°C. Slides were mounted in Vectashield anti-fade medium with DAPI (Vector Laboratories #H-1500) to detect cell nuclei.

Quantification

Immunofluorescence, CHP, and EBD images were visualized using an EVOS M7000 imaging system and software at 10x or 20x magnification (indicated by scale bars). Image brightness and contrast were edited using Adobe Photoshop, keeping edits consistent across experimental replicates. For percent positive cell quantifications, total number of cell nuclei and then total number of positive cells in both left and right leaflets were counted using ImageJ v1.53 [155]. Number of positive cells was calculated as a percentage of total valve cells. For corrected total cell fluorescence (CTCF) measurements, average background fluorescence from each image was subtracted from the integrated density (a measurement of pixel intensity normalized to area) of the selected fluorescent channel in the AoV region as measured by ImageJ to calculate average CTCF for each image. Statistical analysis was performed in GraphPad Prism 9.0 as indicated in corresponding figure legends.

3.2.6 RNA-Sequencing

Tissue Collection and RNA-Sequencing

AoVs from wild type young and aging *c57BL/6J* mice were isolated 48 hours after AoV wire injury with minimal myocardial contamination and immediately flash frozen in liquid nitrogen. Each group consisted of a biological n of 3 with one AoV per biological n. Frozen samples were sent to Ocean Ridge Biosciences LLC (Palm Gardens Beach, FL), where RNA isolation and sequencing was performed as follows.

Total RNA was isolated from the tissue samples using TRI Reagent according to the manufacturer's user manual (Molecular Research Center #TR118). Following isolation, RNA was quantified by O.D. measurement, digested with RNase free DNase I (Epicentre #D9905K), and re-purified using RNA Clean XP magnetic beads (Beckman Coulter #A63987). The newly digested RNA samples were then assessed by denaturing gel electrophoresis using a 1% agarose – 2 % formaldehyde gel.

Amplified cDNA libraries suitable for sequencing were prepared from 200 nanograms (ng) of DNA-free total RNA using the Universal Plus mRNA-Seq Library Prep Kit (NuGEN Technologies, Inc. #0508-96). The quality and size distribution of the amplified libraries were determined by chip-based capillary electrophoresis on Agilent

2100 Bioanalyzer High Sensitivity DNA assays (Agilent Technologies #5067-4626). Libraries were quantified using the Takara Library Quantification Kit (#638324).

The libraries were pooled at equimolar concentrations and diluted prior to loading onto a flow-cell on an Illumina cBot. The libraries were extended, and bridge amplified to create sequence clusters. The flow cell was transferred to the HiSeq 4000 instrument and sequenced using 150 nt paired-end reads plus a single index read.

Raw FASTQs were split into files containing 4,000,000 reads and checked for quality using the FASTX-Toolkit. The reads were filtered (removing sequences that did not pass Illumina's quality filter) and trimmed based on the quality results (3 nucleotides at the left end of the R1 reads and 1nt at the left end of the R2 reads). Sequence alignment was performed using TopHat v2.1.0 to the mm10 genome. BAM files were merged on a per sample. Exon and gene level counting were performed using the easyRNASeq version 2.4.7 package. A binary annotation file, built using the annotation file generation function of EasyRNASeq, was used for this analysis; the Ensembl release 83 GTF file was used as input. Annotation was performed using a Gene Transfer Format (GTF) annotation file for Mus musculus which contains the current Ensembl Mouse release 83. Filtering of the reads per kilobase million (RPKM) values was performed to retain a list of genes with a minimum of approximately 50 mapped reads in 25% or more samples. The threshold of 50 mapped reads is considered the Reliable Quantification Threshold, as the RPKM values for a gene represented by 50 reads should be reproducible in technical replicates. To avoid reporting large fold changes due to random variation of counts from low abundance mRNA, RPKM values equivalent to a count of <= 10 reads per gene were replaced with the average RPKM value equivalent to 10 reads/gene across all the samples in the experiment.

A two-way ANOVA was performed to identify genes that differed significantly in their expression levels due to Age or Surgery. The filtered and adjusted RPKM data for 13,526 nuclear protein-coding mouse genes with detectable RNA expression were used as input for this analysis. Post-hoc Tukey Tests were then calculated to determine genes that significantly differed between Ages within each Surgery condition and between each Surgery condition within each Age group. Fold changes were also calculated and reported for the same comparisons as the Turkey Tests using the mean of each group being compared. If the average of both groups in a comparison fell below the average of their respective detection thresholds (RQT), then 'NA' was reported. False discovery rates (FDR) were calculated by the method of Benjamini and Hochberg [156]. All statistical analysis was performed using R computing software version 3.2.2.

PCA Analysis

Principal Component Analysis (PCA) was performed on the RPKM data for all 13,526 detectable (>= RQT in at least 25% of the samples) nuclear protein-coding mouse genes. The RPKM values were log10-transformed, centered so that each sample had mean 0, and the first three principal components were calculated. To find genes that substantially contribute to each PC value, the correlation and fold-change in expression of each gene with the first three principal components was calculated according to the methods of Sharov et al. [157]. Genes with a positive or negative correlation of at least 0.9 and a fold change of at least 1.7 compared with the principal components are reported.

Hierarchical Clustering

RPKM data for 13,526 nuclear protein-coding genes with detectable mRNA levels was used for hierarchical clustering analysis by Cluster 3.0 software [158]. Genes were median centered prior to hierarchical clustering. Hierarchical clustering was conducted using centered correlation as the similarity metric and average linkage as the clustering method. Along with clustering gene expressions was shown based on supplied sample grouping in the form of a heatmap for the genes with a Tukey FDR < 0.1.

Bubble Plot, Circle Plot, and Chord Plot

Functional annotation was performed on genes differentially expressed between injury (n=3) and sham (n=3) groups with a false discovery rate (FDR) < 0.2, to correct for multiple testing. 96 genes were considered to be differentially expressed and were analyzed using the Database for Annotation, Visualization and Integrated Discovery (DAVID) v6.8 [114, 159]. Gene Ontology (GO) Direct terms were examined, which provide GO mappings directly annotated by the source database, and included Biological Processes (BP), Cellular Components (CC), and Molecular Functions (MF). GOplot v1.0.2 was utilized to visualize the GO annotations, and all analysis was performed with Rv4.0.3 [160]. The z-score was calculated by GOplot and is used to predict the overall expression change of a GOterm. The equation is as follows, where up and down are the number of assigned genes up-regulated (logFC>0) in the data or down- regulated (logFC<0):

$$zscore = \frac{(up - down)}{\sqrt{count}}$$

6-well tissue culture plates were coated with 0.15µg/ml type 1 rat tail collagen (Corning #354236) in 1xPBS for 1 hour at 37°C before aspirating remaining collagen solution and rinsing with 1xPBS. Plates were then seeded with primary porcine valve endothelial cells (pAVECs) in DMEM (Corning #10-017-CV) supplemented with 2% fetal bovine serum (FBS) and 0.275mg/ml heparin (Sigma-Aldrich #H4784). After reaching confluency, a scratch was created in the middle of each well using a p1000 pipette tip, or no scratch was created for the control wells. 1 or 2 hours post-scratch, cells were fixed with 4% paraformaldehyde/1xPBS for 15 minutes at room temperature before permeabilization with 0.25% triton-X 100 (Sigma-Aldrich #T9284) in 1xPBS. Cells were then incubated with rabbit α pSmad2 primary antibody (Invitrogen #44-244, 1:200) overnight at 4°C. For primary antibody detection, cells were incubated with Alexa Fluor 594 donkey α rabbit secondary antibody (LifeTechnologies, 1:400) for 1 hour at room temperature before mounting with Vectashield anti-fade medium with DAPI (Vector Laboratories #H-1500) to detect cell nuclei.

Quantification of pSmad2 Images

Images of pSmad2 immunofluorescence were visualized using an EVOS M7000 imaging system and software at either 10x or 20x magnification (indicated by scale bars). Image brightness and contrast were edited using Adobe Photoshop, keeping edits consistent across experimental replicates. Using ImageJ, total pSmad2 levels were quantified by total CTCF in the red channel for each field, and then normalized to the number of DAPI-positive nuclei per field to give the amount of pSmad2 per cell. To calculate nuclear levels of pSmad2, DAPI-positive nuclei were detected and outlined in ImageJ to create a region of interest which was then applied to the red channel, and intensity within the region of interest was measured, then normalized to the total number of DAPI-positive nuclei. Statistical analysis was performed in GraphPad Prism 9.0 as indicated in corresponding figure legend.

3.2.8 Tgfβ1 Treatment Assay

Treatment

Primary porcine aortic valve interstitial cells (pAVICS) were plated in 6 well plates in DMEM (Corning #10-017-CV) supplemented with 2% FBS. When cells reached approximately 70% confluency, media was aspirated and replaced with fresh media supplemented with Tgfβ1 (Sigma-Aldrich #H8541) at a final in-well concentration of 10ng/ml or 1xPBS for control wells.

RNA Isolation and qRT-PCR

24 hours after Tgfβ1 treatment, RNA was isolated from each well as previously described. Briefly, 1ml of TRIzol (Thermo Fisher #15596018) was added to each well and incubated for 5 minutes at room temperature before pipetting into a clean tube. 200µl of chloroform was added and incubated on ice for 5 minutes before centrifuging at 14,000 RCF for 30 minutes at 4°C. The top layer containing the RNA was then transferred to a clean tube and RNA precipitated using 400µl isopropanol and centrifuging at 14,000 RCF for 20 minutes to form a pellet. The RNA pellet was washed twice in ice cold 70% ethanol,

dried, and resuspended in nuclease-free water. RNA concentration was determined using a NanoDrop 2000.

cDNA for each sample was synthesized from 200ng of RNA using the High-Capacity RNA-to-cDNA kit (Applied Biosystems #4387406). Quantitative real-time PCR (qRT-PCR) was performed with Fast SYBR Green master mix (Applied Biosystems #4385612) and probes designed to detect porcine *Cthrc1* with forward sequence 5' CCG GTC GGG ATG GAT TCA AA 3' and reverse sequence 5' CCG AG TGA GCC ACT GAA CA 3'. A StepOnePlus Real-Time PCR System (Applied Biosystems) was used to detect changes in gene expression. Cycle counts for each target gene were normalized to *18s* expression, and differences in gene expression were reported as a fold change from the untreated condition. Statistical analysis was performed in GraphPad Prism 9.0.

3.3 Results

3.3.1 Valve Endothelial Barrier Function is Restored by 48hr After Damage by Wire Injury

Injury, damage, or dysfunction of the valve endothelium is considered to be an initiating step of valve disease, but there are few model systems available to examine this. Therefore, the goal of this study was to modify a previously established model of wire-induced AoV injury [76], but reduce the severity of insult and subsequently examine the short-term response in the absence of the induction of a severe pathological program. The surgical wire injury model was performed in adult (2-3 month old) wild type (WT) mice (Fig. 7A) by inserting a 0.36mm angioplasty guidewire into the carotid artery and advancing it through the AoV opening under echocardiographic guidance (Fig. 7B). The wire was moved in and out across the valve opening in a "scratching" motion, then positioned inside the left ventricle and "spun" on the surface of the AoV. The original model repeated these motions over 50 times each with the intent of provoking severe damage, while our adapted model included only 20 of each motion. These adjustments effectively reduced the total level of injury, as suggested by the lack of inflammatory response, calcification, and ECM changes.

To confirm that this mild wire injury approach was sufficient to induce endothelial injury, permeability of the VEC layer was quantified as an indicator of endothelial damage and dysfunction. Changes in endothelial permeability were examined by injecting Evans Blue Dye (EBD) into the circulation, where it was able to distribute and penetrate any permeable barrier, including the injured valve endothelium. EBD infiltration into the AoV was examined at 6 hours, 48 hours, and 4 weeks post-surgery in order to analyze barrier function throughout the short-term response to endothelial injury (Fig. 7C and D).

In sham controls, low levels of EBD were able to cross the valve endothelium, indicating minimal damage at all timepoints. At 6 hours post-injury, EBD intensity within the AoV cusps increased almost 2-fold compared to sham controls (Fig. 7D), demonstrating increased endothelial permeability as a result of the wire injury procedure. However, EBD intensity within the AoV at 48 hours post-injury was comparable to the level seen in sham controls (Fig. 7C and D), implying a lower level of endothelial permeability. This low level of EBD infiltration into the injured AoV was maintained at 4 weeks post-injury (Fig. 7C and D). These data suggest initial damage to the endothelial layer is occurring by 6 hours post-injury, but that barrier function is restored by 48 hours post-injury.

Previous studies have shown an association between VEC damage or injury, and pathological ECM disturbances of the valve cups [68-72]. To investigate potential disruptions in matrix quantity or organization as a result of mild wire injury damage, ECM components of the valve were examined. Fibrillar collagen, present in the fibrosa layer of the healthy valve, was visualized and quantified using a collagen hybridizing peptide (CHP) (Fig. 7E). As shown, CHP immunoreactivity revealed no change in overall collagen levels in the AoV at 4 weeks post-surgery (Fig. 7F). In contrast, cleaved versican, suggestive of active ECM remodeling was also examined (Fig. 7G) and shown to be significantly increased at 4 weeks post-injury (Fig. 7H). However, these subtle changes in the ECM as a result of endothelial damage did not evoke significant functional impairment (data not shown) within the 4 week time period examined.

3.3.2 RNA-Sequencing Reveals Involvement of Proliferation and Extracellular Matrix Signaling in the Valve Endothelial Injury Response

To better understand the observed restoration of the endothelial layer (Fig. 7C and D) at the molecular level, bulk RNA-sequencing was performed on injured and sham AoV isolated 48 hours post-surgery. Hierarchical heat map analysis (Fig. 8A) and PCA clustering analysis (Fig. 8B) revealed similarities between replicates in sham and injured groups indicating a clear transcriptional profile associated with the valve response to endothelial injury and restoration of barrier function. Gene ontology (GO) analysis was performed in order to categorize the transcripts which were most significantly differentially expressed between injury and sham valves. The top 20 GO terms (Fig. 8C) included many terms related to cell proliferation including mitotic nuclear division, cell division, and cell cycle. GO terms relating to the ECM were also highly differentially expressed, including collagen trimer, extracellular matrix, proteinaceous extracellular matrix, and collagen biosynthetic process. A closer analysis of the expression patterns in each GO term (Fig. 8D) revealed that the top 12 terms were all upregulated in injured compared sham valves, indicating that the injury response process involves increased signaling and coordination of many pathways but especially those involved in cell proliferation and ECM remodeling. Common proliferation-related and valve ECM genes and their relationship to the respective GO terms in shown in Fig. 8E.

3.3.3 Proliferation of Multiple Endogenous Cell Types Occurs in Response to Valve Endothelial Injury

Based on GO profiling indicating significant upregulation of mitosis and cell cycle-related transcripts in injured valves, valve cell proliferation was examined at 48 hours post-surgery to validate RNA-seq findings, as well as at 6 hours and 4 weeks in order to explore proliferation throughout the short-term response to AoV endothelial injury. Phospho-histone H3 (pHH3) immunofluorescence was utilized as a marker of active cell proliferation (Fig. 9A). Quantification of pHH3 immunoreactivity indicated a dramatic increase in the percentage of proliferating cells in the injured AoV 6 hours post-surgery with approximately 8% of valve cells proliferating, compared to about 1% proliferation in sham controls (Fig. 9B). The level of proliferation in injured valves decreased to approximately 3% by 48 hours post-injury, and returned to baseline sham levels by 4 weeks-post injury.

To determine which cell types were proliferating following valve endothelial injury, co-staining of pHH3 was performed with endothelial (VE-cadherin) and immune (CD45) cell markers. At 6 hours post-injury, 8% of valve cells were pHH3-positive, and 40.04% of these were also positive for endothelial marker VE-cadherin (Fig. 9C and D), demonstrating the presence of actively proliferating endothelial cells. At this same timepoint, 25.13% of pHH3-positive cells co-stained with immune marker CD45 (Fig. 9E and F), revealing that the immune cell population is also actively proliferating. By 48 hours post-injury, overall cell proliferation decreased to just over 3%, but 45.81% of these pHH3-positive cells remained positive for VE-cadherin (Fig. 9D) and 52.73% remained CD45-positive (Fig. 9F). A population of pHH3-positive cells negative for both VE-cadherin or CD45 comprised approximately 25%-50% of proliferating cells at each timepoint (Fig. 9C and E). These cells are presumed to be VICs and are likely contributing to active proliferation as well.

Although both VE-cadherin-positive and CD45-positive cell populations demonstrated proliferative capacity, the overall percentage of VE-cadherin-positive (Fig. 9G) and CD45-positive (Fig. 9H) cells were unchanged in the AoV as a function of injury or time. The total number of cells per valve also remained unchanged (data not shown). These results suggest that multiple sub-populations of cell lineages within the cusp undergo proliferation within 6 hours and continue to proliferate at lower levels up to 48 hours post-endothelial injury.

3.3.4 Cthrc1 and Tgfβ1 are Involved in the Valve Injury Response

An in-depth examination of ECM-related signaling in the RNA-sequencing data revealed a 6.65-fold increase in post-injury expression of collagen triple helix repeat containing 1 (*Cthrc1*) transcript, although baseline sham expression levels were low (Fig. 10A). To validate increased post-injury levels of Cthrc1 at the protein level, immunofluorescence was performed on 48 hour post-surgery AoV sections (Fig. 10B). Quantification of protein immunoreactivity (Fig. 10C) confirmed a significant increase in post-injury levels of Cthrc1, and localization studies suggest enrichment within the interstitium, consistent with the known role of Cthrc1 in fibroblast-like cells following injury (Fig. 10B) [161-164]. Cthrc1 is also known to be regulated upstream by canonical Tgfβ1 signaling [161, 165-167] and RNA-seq analysis shows a 1.47-fold increase in *Tgfβ1* transcript 48 hours post-injury (Fig. 10D). Additional immunofluorescence confirmed increased Tgfβ1 protein with apparent enrichment in the endothelial region (Fig. 10E and F), where it is known to be expressed in healthy valves [22].

To more clearly explore the Tgfβ1-Cthrc1 signaling axis, *in vitro* experiments were performed to determine if injury to the valve endothelium results in an upregulation of canonical Tgfβ1 activity. Accordingly, confluent porcine aortic valve endothelial cells (pAVECs) were subjected to scratch injury or left uninjured as a control condition, and expression and localization of phospo-Smad2 (pSmad2) was examined by immunofluorescence at 1 and 2 hours post-injury as a measure of canonical Tgfβ1 activity (Fig. 11A). Total (nuclear and cytoplasmic) pSmad2 immunoreactivity was measured (Fig. 11B), along with nuclear intensity alone (Fig. 11C) as an indicator of active Tgfβ1 signaling. Quantification revealed over 40% higher total pSmad2 levels 1 hour after injury as compared to uninjured controls, while nuclear pSmad2 levels increased by over 45%. This increase in pSmad2 level and activity after pAVEC injury suggests that canonical Tgfβ1 signaling pathway is activated in response to VEC damage.

To next examine whether Tgfβ1 activity can lead to increased expression of Cthrc1 in VICs as observed *in vivo* (Fig. 10B), pAVICs were treated with 10ng/ml Tgfβ1 for 24 hours and *Cthrc1* RNA levels were measured. Quantitative real-time PCR (qRT-PCR) results confirmed an approximate 2-fold increase in *Cthrc1* expression in Tgfβ1-treated pAVICs compared to untreated controls (Fig. 11D). These results together suggest that the mechanistic response to AoV endothelial damage and the subsequent restoration of the endothelial barrier may involve a Tgfβ1-Cthrc1 signaling axis.

3.3.5 Injured Cthrc1$^{-/-}$ *Mice Display a Decreased Capacity to Restore Endothelial Barrier Function*

Cthrc1 has been shown to play a role in the response to tissue injury in other organ systems and is known to promote cell proliferation and wound healing [161, 165, 168, 169], and our data shows a similar association in injured valves. To determine the requirement for Cthrc1 in the cell proliferation and endothelial barrier restoration observed after VEC damage, the wire injury procedure was performed in *Cthrc1$^{-/-}$* mice. Proliferation was examined by pHH3 staining 48 hours post-injury in *Cthrc1$^{-/-}$* mice and WT littermates (Fig. 12A). Quantification reveals a non-significant trend towards a decreased proliferative index in *Cthrc1$^{-/-}$* mice, with an average of 26% lower pHH3-positive cells in injured *Cthrc1$^{-/-}$* AoV compared to injured WT littermates (Fig. 12B). EBD endothelial permeability experiments (Fig. 12C) revealed a similar pattern, with injured WT littermates exhibiting permeability 1.8 times higher than in shams, while injured *Cthrc1-/-* mice show a 3.9-fold increase in EBD infiltration compared to infiltration in respective sham controls (Fig. 12D), although these differences do not reach statistical significance with the current number of replicates. These preliminary results indicate that Cthrc1 deficiency impairs restoration of the endothelial barrier after damage, potentially through reduction of proliferative capacity.

3.3.6 A Proposed Model for Valve Response to Endothelial Damage

Based on the results described, a potential hypothesis for the AoV response to endothelial damage was proposed (Fig. 13). In this model, endothelial damage leads to upregulated endothelial Tgfβ1 signaling indicated by the presence of increased pSmad2. This VEC-derived Tgfβ1 then leads to an increase in interstitial production of Cthrc1, which in turn leads to higher rates of total valve cell proliferation and restoration of the endothelial barrier.

3.3.7 Aging Adult Mice Demonstrate Decreased Repair Capacity in Response to Valve Endothelial Injury

The risk of valve disease development is known to increase with advanced age [65], and it has also been shown that aging in mice leads to a decline in VEC function and barrier integrity [60]. To examine how these factors influence the response to endothelial damage, the wire injury procedure was performed in aging adult (16-18 month old) mice, and RNA-sequencing was performed in parallel with the previously described studies in younger adult mice.

Despite the post-injury increases observed in healthy adult mice, RNA-sequencing results revealed no significant increase in *Tgfβ1* (Fig. 14A) or *Cthrc1* (Fig. 14B) transcript in the aging adult AoV 48 hours post-injury. Protein levels as measured by immunofluorescence follow a similar trend, with Tgfβ1 levels comparable to sham controls (Fig. 14C and D), and Cthrc1 exhibiting a lower level of increased expression than that seen in healthy adults (Fig. 14E and F).

To examine the association of decreased post-injury Tgfβ1 and Cthrc1 levels with proliferative capacity, pHH3 immunoreactivity was also examined in aging adult mice post-injury (Fig. 15A). Although a proliferation rate of 1.96% was observed in aging adult mice at 48 hours post-surgery, this percentage is significantly lower than the 3.19% seen in healthy adult mice (Fig. 15B). This decreased proliferative capacity may translate to a diminished or delayed ability to repair the endothelial barrier, as indicated by a 1.5-fold higher EBD intensity in the aging adult AoV compared to sham controls at 4 weeks post-surgery (Fig. 15C and D).

This data in aging adult mice provides additional evidence for the relationship between the Tgfβ1-Cthrc1 signaling axis and proliferation and subsequent restoration of the valve endothelium. These experiments also demonstrate a potential rationale for the increased risk of valve disease development in the aging population due to a decreased capacity to restore endothelial barrier function after injury.

3.4 Discussion

Histological investigations of end-stage human valve disease samples have frequently implied an association with valve endothelial damage [75, 150]. Experimental mouse models have more clearly elucidated this connection by demonstrating that genetically targeting VEC function can directly result in pathological changes to valve ECM organization and composition [26, 58]. These studies together suggest that injury or dysfunction of the valve endothelium is an initiating factor in valve disease onset and subsequent progression [68]. Despite this evidence, the potential for therapeutic repair or restoration of the valve endothelial barrier has not been examined as an alternative to the standard treatment of valve replacement surgery. To explore the potential for valve endothelial repair, we adapted a non-genetic surgical model [76] to induce mild injury to the valve endothelium in the absence of severe inflammation or acute disease onset. Utilizing this surgical model, we have identified a beneficial short-term response to mild injury which led to restoration of the damaged endothelial layer within 48 hours. Additional transcriptomics analysis and subsequent *in vivo* and *in vitro* confirmation demonstrated that restoration involves increased endothelial production of Tgfβ1, and higher levels of Cthrc1 within the interstitial compartment. In association with these molecular changes, cell proliferation is significantly increased in multiple native valve cell populations which likely contribute to the beneficial reparative response. In contrast to healthy adults, aging adults with pre-existing endothelial dysfunction [60] did not possess the ability to restore the injured valve endothelium. Overall, this investigation highlights the endogenous repair potential of the healthy adult valve endothelium and explores elements of the mechanisms responsible for this therapeutically relevant response to VEC damage.

In adult cardiac valves, Tgfβ1 is secreted by VECs and is known to be an important signaling mediator to prevent development of valve disease [25, 170, 171]. Here, we observe elevated levels of Tgfβ1 in the endothelial region of the AoV in injured valves compared to sham controls (Fig. 10E), and show increased signaling in response to damage in cultured VECs (Fig. 11). These results suggest that although baseline expression is required during normal valve homeostasis, levels of Tgfβ1 increase as a feature of the endothelial injury response. In other injured tissues, Cthrc1 has been shown to play an important role in the essential proliferation and migration aspects of wound healing [161, 163, 165, 168, 169]. Studies have indicated that Cthrc1 is largely secreted from fibroblast or smooth muscle cell types in response to injury [163, 169], consistent with our data showing enrichment of Cthrc1 expression within the interstitial region of the valve occupied by fibroblast-like VICs (Fig. 10B). Analysis in other systems has shown that Cthrc1 can be both positively and negatively regulated upstream by Tgfβ1 [161, 162, 167], however in our *in vitro* system we observe a positive regulation in VICs following endogenous Tgfβ1 treatment. Additionally, our *in vivo* data showing a reciprocal increase in both Tgfβ1 and Cthrc1 after wire injury also indicates a positive regulatory relationship. Together, these results suggest that in response to mild injury, endothelial-derived secreted Tgfβ1 acts in a paracrine manner to stimulate Cthrc1 expression in VICs. However, comprehensive cell specific knockout models will be important for more closely examining the requirement of these signals in VECs and VICs during the repair response.

Previously, Cthrc1 has been shown to induce both proliferation and cell migration [163, 165, 168]. Cthrc1 is upstream of the MAPK pathway and is specifically involved in the phosphorylation status of ERK1/2, which subsequently activates Fos related antigen 1 (Fra1). When active, Fra1 functions as a transcription factor and can promote production of cyclin D1 to directly induce cell cycle progression and proliferation [165, 172]. Although the phosphorylation and activation statuses of ERK1/2 and Fra1 have yet to be determined in our model, we do observe a significant 1.59-fold increase in *Ccnd1* (cyclin D1) expression following damage to the endothelium, suggesting a potential conservation of this pathway in native valve cell types. While the requirement of Cthrc1 to promote valve cell proliferation after endothelial injury has yet to be confirmed, preliminary data from *Cthrc1*[-/-] mice are encouraging, as injured mice exhibit a lower proliferative index post-injury compared to WT littermates (Fig. 12A and B). In addition to promoting *Ccnd1* expression, Cthrc1-mediated Fra1 is also known to upregulate Mmp14 (matrix metalloproteinase 14), a recognized regulator of cell migration [172-174]. Mmp14 may act to remodel the ECM by degrading various components and allowing cells to move more freely within the matrix-rich valve structure. RNA-sequencing analysis shows a significant 2.23-fold increase in *Mmp14* expression in injured valves, suggesting that this mechanism of cell migration might allow for the physical movement of existing valve cells to restore the damaged endothelium. However, future studies utilizing the Cthrc1 loss of function model are needed in order to confirm the precise pathway which links post-injury upregulation of Cthrc1 to proliferation and migration of the valve cell types observed here.

Within the short-term response to endothelial injury, we observe a significant increase in proliferation of multiple native valve cell types, including VE-cadherin-positive endothelial cells, CD45-positive immune cells, and a third population negative for these markers (likely VIC-associated). At both 6 and 48 hours post-injury, proliferating endothelial cells make up approximately 40-45% of the total proliferating population (Fig.

9D), indicating uniform contribution throughout the short-term injury response. As seen in studies of vascular endothelial injury, proliferation and subsequent migration of neighboring undamaged endothelial cells directly contribute to replace or replenish the damaged endothelium [98]. Based on our data, we hypothesize that similar mechanisms may underlie the reparative response in the valves, potentially mediated by Tgfβ1-Cthrc1 signaling. In spite of the observed endothelial proliferation, the total number of VE-cadherin-positive endothelial cells stays constant through the examined timepoints (Fig. 9G). This could suggest several possibilities, including an overall balance between cell death and proliferation, a lack of total proliferating cell engraftment, or the transformation of endothelial cells via endothelial to mesenchymal transition (endMT) [49]. However, molecular indicators of newly transformed mesenchyme cells, such as increased smooth muscle alpha actin (α-SMA), were not detected by RNA-sequencing or immunohistochemistry following injury.

We also identified a proliferative contribution from CD45-positive cells, a large portion of which are adjacent to the endothelial barrier (Fig. 9E). This immune population constitutes approximately 25% of the proliferating cells at 6 hours post-injury, but by 48 hours post-injury increases to almost 53% (Fig. 9F), suggesting a biphasic response. However, similar to the endothelial population, the total number of CD45-positive cells in the valve does not increase throughout the short-term response period observed (Fig. 9H), indicating the absence of extensive CD45-positive cell infiltration. The precise role of CD45-positive cells in the context of valve injury remains to be examined. However, previous work in diseased valves suggests that resident CD45-positive cells secrete chemokines and potentially mediate ECM remodeling [175, 176], while studies in the myocardium following injury report immune cell-mediated release of chemokines and additional factors to promote the recovery process [177, 178].

Proliferating cells negative for both CD45 and VE-cadherin were also observed in the injured valve. Based on the lack of marker expression and the interstitial localization, these cells are likely VICs and may passively proliferate in response to the secreted Cthrc1 signal. However, to fully appreciate the nuances of post-injury AoV cell proliferation and resulting endothelial barrier restoration, lineage tracing and fate mapping studies will be required. Tracing molecular profiles of single cells during the restoration process would also contribute to our understanding of the cell-specific responses to endothelial damage and would help determine the identities and functions of cells which directly contribute to restoring the injured endothelial barrier.

Aging has been linked to VEC dysfunction and is associated with susceptibility to valve disease [60, 65]. Interestingly, our data shows that aging adult mice have limited capacity to respond to the endothelial injury created by the wire injury procedure. This is associated with attenuated increases in Tgfβ1 and Cthrc1 and a reduced proliferative index (Fig. 14 and 15). As an associated consequence, the endothelial barrier in aging adult mice remained permeable in EBD experiments even at 4 weeks post-injury (Fig. 15C and D). Multiple factors could contribute to the reduced mechanistic response in aging adult mice. Existing baseline levels of VEC dysfunction in aging adult mice, as demonstrated by our lab [60], could prevent the AoV from generating a strong and sufficient response to injury. It is also well-established that cells lose proliferative and signaling capacity as they age

[179, 180], and accordingly the aging AoV cells may be incapable of creating or responding to the restorative signals which occur in the healthy adult valve. An important next step will involve investigating the possibility of exogenously upregulating the described Tgfβ1-Cthrc1 mechanism in aging mice and additional valve disease models with known VEC dysfunction. This will allow for exploration into the potential to prevent or slow valve disease progression by introduction of the beneficial response observed in healthy adult mice.

This study has demonstrated that in mice, the healthy adult AoV is able to restore endothelial function after damage to the endothelium, and that the injury response and restoration process involves a molecular VEC-VIC signaling cascade. Additionally, the data described here indicates that multiple cell types in the valve maintain proliferative capacity even in adult stages. This has also recently been demonstrated in a zebrafish cell ablation model which illustrated the involvement of a variety of proliferating cell types in the adult zebrafish regeneration of the AV valve [100, 181]. Interestingly, we do observe some mechanistic response and proliferation ability in aging adult valves. Although this response occurs at a lower overall level insufficient to promote endothelial repair, these results may provide evidence that even aging valves retain some minimal capacity to respond to damage when stimulated. Clinically, this data implies the existence of an active process which allows for endogenous repair of the valve endothelium but may decline with age. As VEC signaling and barrier function are crucial for promoting VIC maintenance of a healthy valve ECM [22, 68], these results indicate that therapeutic preservation of the valve endothelium could be a mechanism for sustaining healthy valve structure and function, and specifically that upregulation of the Tgfβ1-Cthrc1 signaling axis described here could promote repair and restoration of the AoV endothelium in the context of damage.

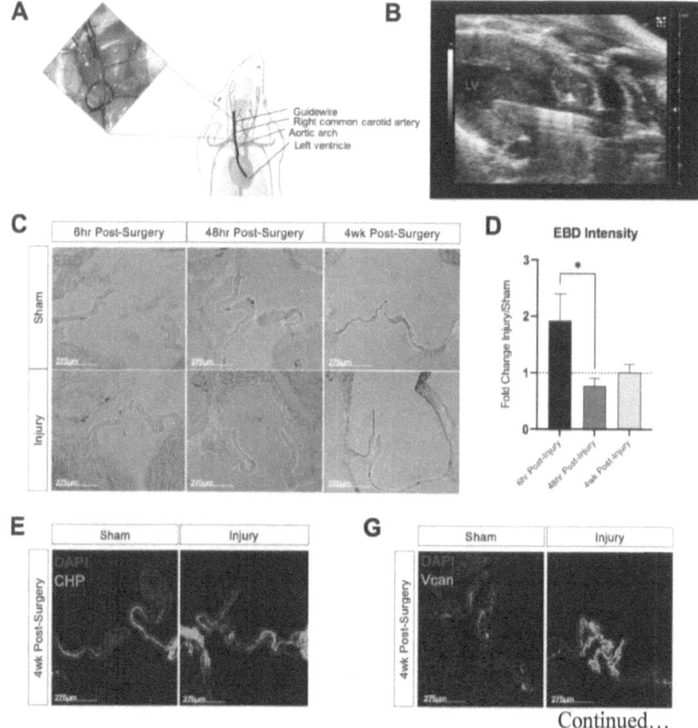

Figure 7: Wire Injury Surgery Causes Endothelial Damage and Possible ECM Remodeling

A) Schematic describing the wire injury surgical procedure. **B)** Echocardiographic image showing wire passing through the AoV. **C)** Evans Blue Dye (EBD) (shown in red) infiltration into injured and sham valves at 6hr, 48hr, and 4wk post-surgery. **D)** Quantification of EBD intensity as a fold change of injured normalized to sham valves. **E)** Collagen hybridizing peptide (CHP) immunofluorescence at 4wk post-surgery. **F)** Quantification of CHP corrected total cell fluorescence (CTCF). **G)** Cleaved versican immunofluorescence at 4wk post-surgery. **H)** Quantification of cleaved versican CTCF. (n=3-6 per group, *:p<0.05, two-tailed unpaired t-test).

Continued…

F 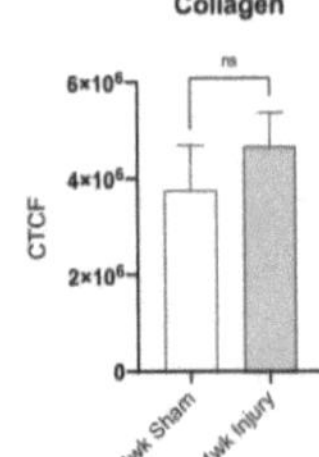

Collagen

H 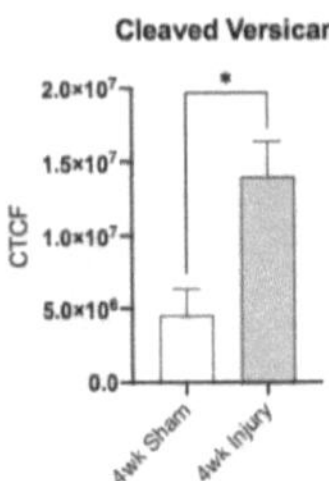

Cleaved Versican

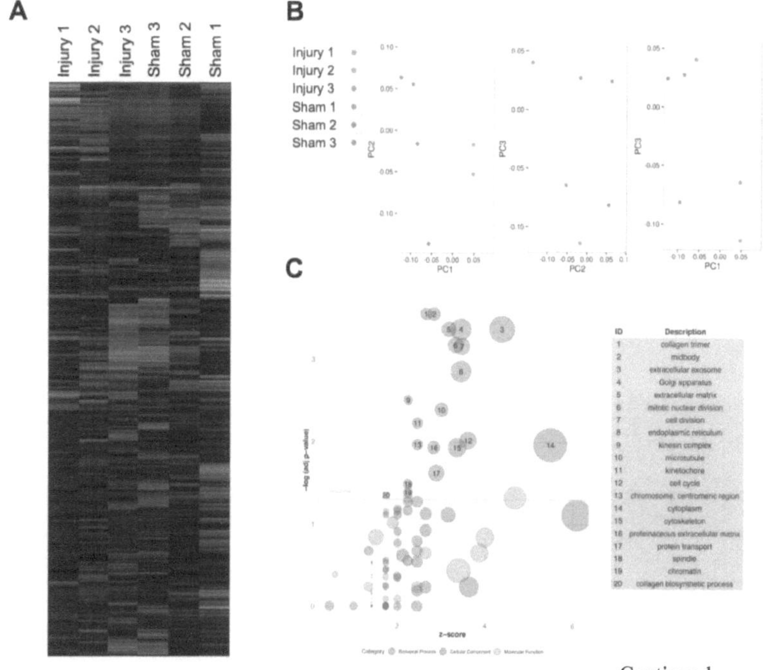

Continued...

Figure 8: RNA-Sequencing Reveals Distinct Post-Injury Transcriptional Profile 48hr After Surgery

A) Hierarchical heatmap cluster showing clustering analysis of biological replicates. **B)** PCA plots showing clustering of biological replicates. **C)** Bubble plot representing gene ontology (GO) terms. Bubble size correlates to number of genes within the term and is plotted based on significance and z-score. Top 20 most significant terms are labeled. Green = biological processes (BP), red = cellular components (CC) and blue = molecular functions (MF). Yellow line represents false discovery rate (FDR) = 0.05. **D)** Circle plot visualizing the top 12 GO terms. Outer circle shows a scatterplot of the genes associated with the term, red = upregulated, blue = downregulated. Inner circle represents FDR by size with larger indicating higher significance and z-score by color with a range from 1.73 (blue) to 5.48 (red). **E)** Chord plot showing 5 GO terms (extracellular matrix, collagen trimer, mitotic nuclear division, cell division and cell cycle) with their relation to 22 significantly differentially expressed genes. Log fold change (logFC) is shown for each gene as a range from 0 (blue) to 1 (red).

Continued…

D
12
11
10
9
8
7
6
5
4
3
2
1
z-score
1.73
5.48
logFC
downregulated
upregulated
ID Description
1   collagen trimer
2   midbody
3   extracellular exosome
4   Golgi apparatus
5   extracellular matrix
6   mitotic nuclear division
7   cell division
8   endoplasmic reticulum
9   kinesin complex
10 microtubule
11 kinetochore
12 cell cycle
E
Extracellular Matrix
Collagen Trimer
Mitotic Nuclear Division
Cell Division
Cell Cycle
logFC
0
1

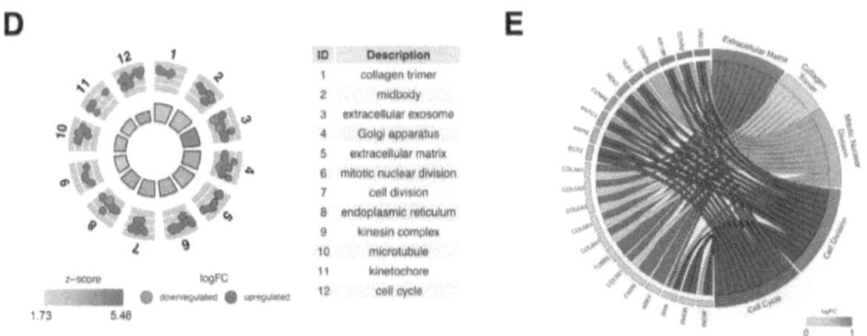

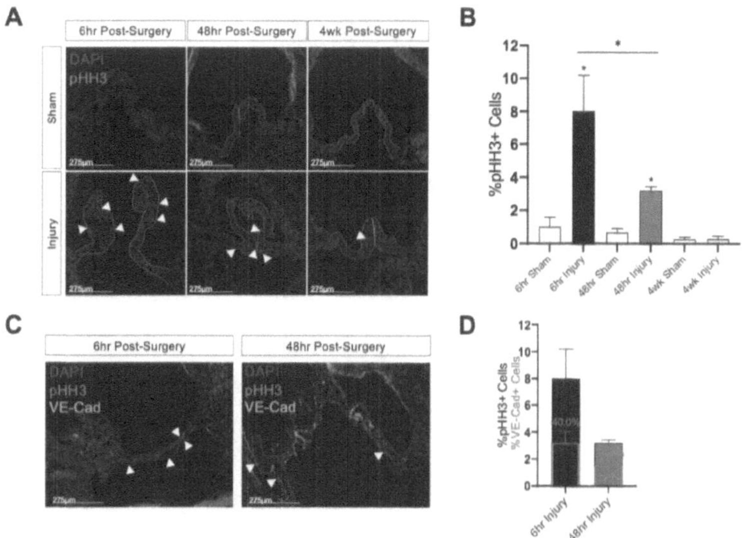

Continued…

Figure 9: Multiple Cell Types Proliferate in Response to Injury

A) Phospho-histone H3 (pHH3) Immunofluorescence in injured and sham valves 6hr, 48hr, and 4wk post-surgery. White arrowheads indicate regions of pHH3-positive cells. **B)** Quantification of the number of pHH3-positive cells as a percentage of the total number of DAPI-labeled nuclei per valve. (*:$p < 0.05$ compared to associated sham control or as indicated by line). **C)** pHH3 and VE-cadherin immunofluorescence in injured valves at 6hr and 48hr post-surgery. White arrowheads indicate double-positive cells. **D)** Quantification of pHH3 and VE-cadherin double positive cells shown as a portion of the total percentage of pHH3-positive cells. **E)** pHH3 and CD45 immunofluorescence in injured valves at 6hr and 48hr post-surgery. White arrowheads indicate regions of double-positive cells. **F)** Quantification of pHH3 and CD45 double positive cells shown as a portion of the total percentage of pHH3-positive cells at each timepoint. **G)** Quantification of VE-cadherin-positive cells as a percentage of the total number of DAPI-labeled nuclei per valve. **H)** Quantification of CD45-positive cells as a percentage of the total number of DAPI-positive nuclei per valve. (n=3-6 per group).

84

Continued…

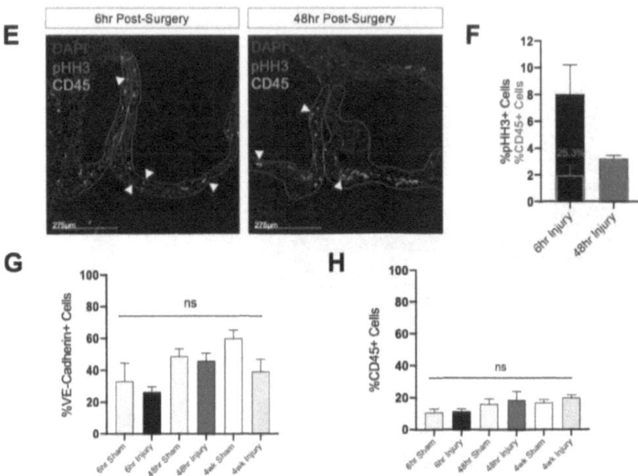

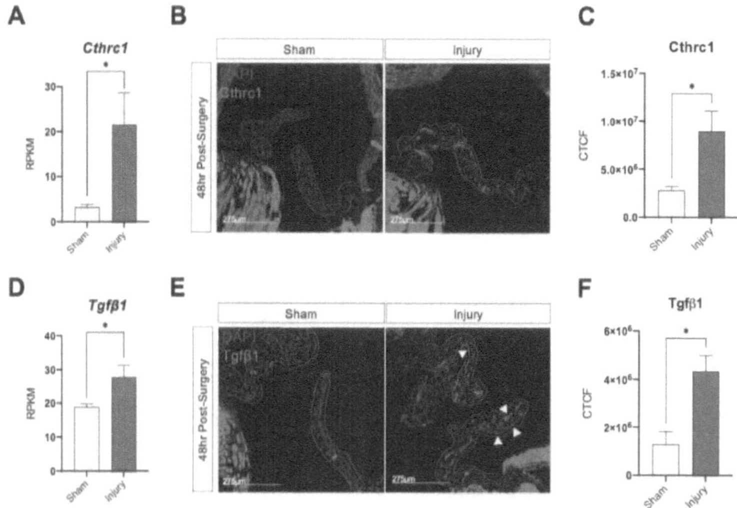

Figure 10: Cthrc1 and Tgfβ1 are Upregulated in Response to Injury

A) *Cthrc1* RPKM levels in injured and sham valves from RNA-seq analysis. **B)** Cthrc1 immunofluorescence in injured and sham valves 48hr post-surgery. **C)** Quantification of Cthrc1 CTCF. **D)** *Tgfβ1* RPKM levels in injured and sham valves from RNA-seq analysis. **E)** Tgfβ1 immunofluorescence in injured and sham valves 48hr post-surgery. White arrowheads indicate areas of endothelial enrichment. **F)** Quantification of Tgfβ1 CTCF. (n=3, *:p<0.05, two-tailed unpaired t test).

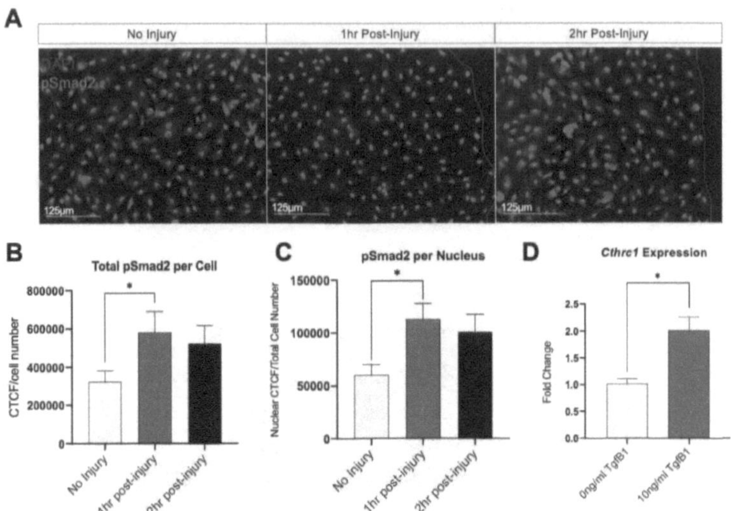

Figure 11: Tgfβ1 and Cthrc1 Signaling in VECs and VICs

A) pSmad2 immunofluorescence in porcine aortic valve endothelial cells (pAVECs) with no injury, 1hr post-injury, and 2hr-post injury. **B)** Quantification of total pSmad2 CTCF over the total number of DAPI-positive nuclei. **C)** Quantification of nuclear pSmad2 CTCF over the total number of DAPI-positive nuclei. **D)** RT-qPCR expression of *Cthrc1* in porcine aortic valve interstitial cells (pAVICS) as a fold change normalized to 0ng/ml Tgfβ1-treated pAVICs. (n=3, *:0<0.05, two-tailed unpaired

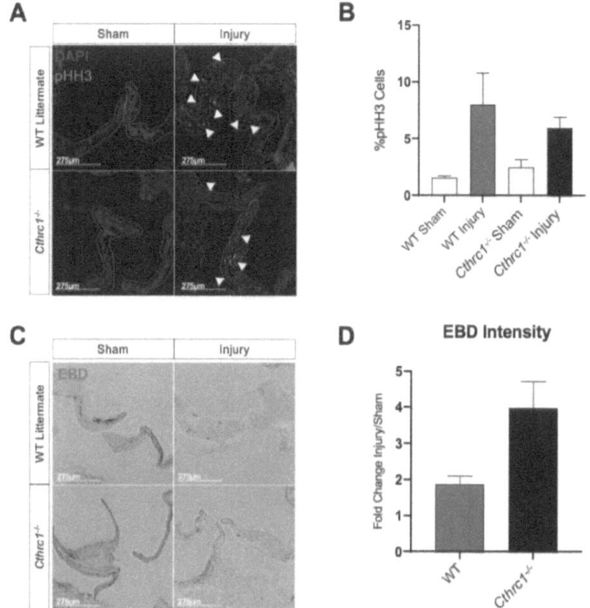

Figure 12: *Cthrc1^{-/-}* Mice Display Potentially Limited Response to Injury

A) pHH3 immunofluorescence in injured and sham WT and *Cthrc1^{-/-}* valves 48hr post-surgery. White arrowheads indicate regions of pHH3-positive cells. **B)** Quantification of the number of pHH3-positive cells as a percentage of the total number of DAPI-labeled nuclei per valve. **C)** EBD infiltration into injured and sham WT and *Cthrc1^{-/-}* valves 48hr post-surgery. **D)** Quantification of EBD intensity as a fold change of injured normalized to sham valves for *Cthrc1^{-/-}* mice and WT littermates. (n=2-3 per group).

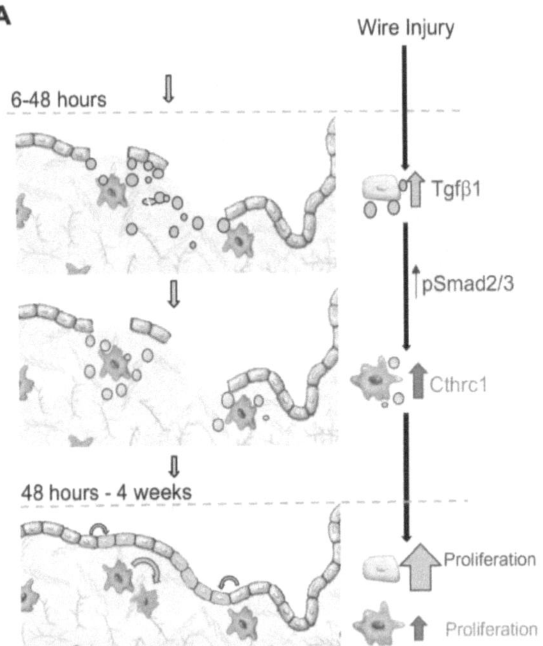

Figure 13: A Proposed Model of AoV Injury Response and Repair

A) Diagram of proposed injury response mechanism, with purple indicating VECs and blue indicating VICs. Initial steps are 6-48hr post-injury while later steps are 48hr-4wk post-injury.

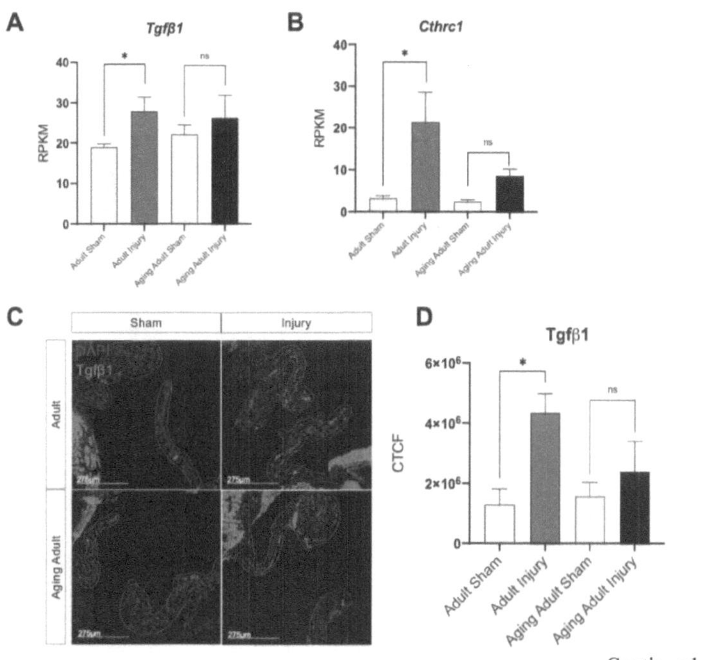

Continued…

Figure 14: Differential Tgfβ1 and Cthrc1 Expression in Aging Adult Mice After Injury

A) *Tgfβ1* RPKM levels in injured and sham valves from adult and aging adult valves. B) *Cthrc1* RPKM levels in injured and sham valves from adult and aging adult valves. C) Tgfβ1 Immunofluorescence 48hr post-injury in adult and aging adult sham and injured valves. **D)** Quantification of Tgfβ1 CTCF. **E)** Cthrc1 immunofluorescence 48hr post-injury in adult and aging adult sham and injured valves. **F)** Quantification of Cthrc1 CTCF. (n=3-6 per group. *:p<0.05 compared to respective sham control, two-tailed unpaired t test).

Continued…

E
Sham
Injury
Adult
Aging Adult
Cthrc1
275μm
275μm
275μm
275μm

F
Cthrc1
1.5×10⁷
1.0×10⁷
5.0×10⁶
0.0
CTCF
*
*
Adult Sham
Adult Injury
Aging Adult Sham
Aging Adult Injury

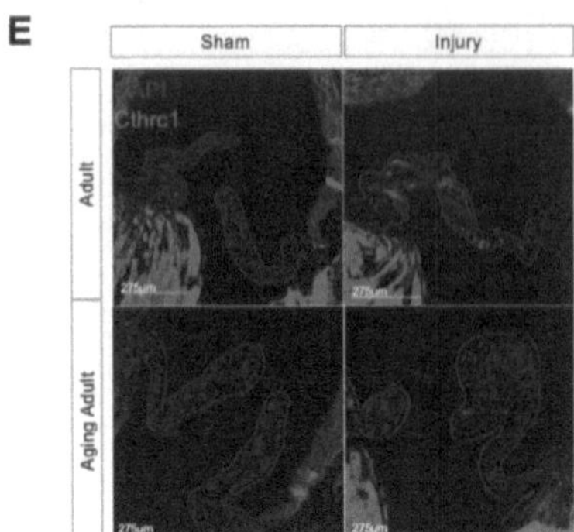

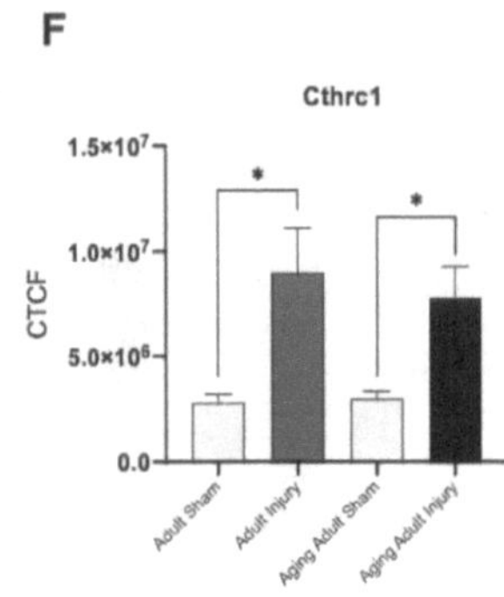

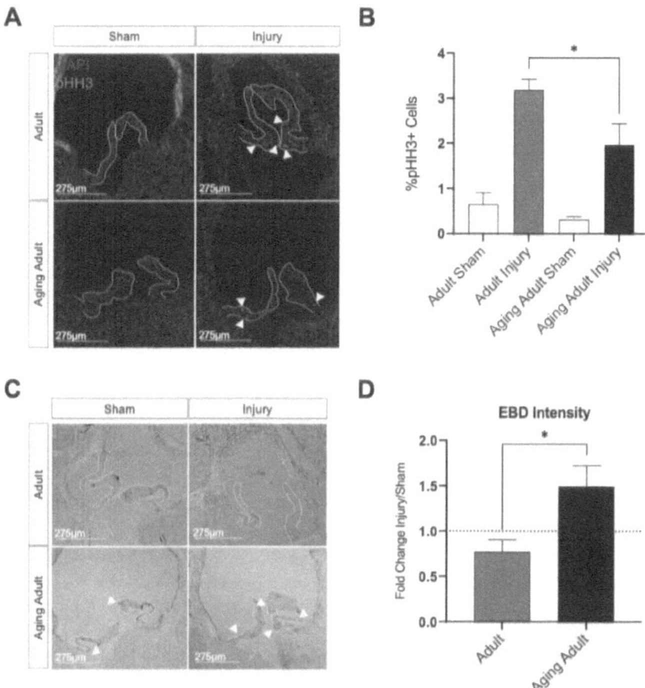

Figure 15: Impaired Repair Response after Injury in Aging Adults

A) pHH3 immunofluorescence 48hr post-injury in adult and aging adult sham and injured valves. White arrowheads indicate regions of pHH3-positive cells. **B)** Quantification of pHH3-positive cells as a percentage of total DAPI-positive nuclei per valve. **C)** EBD infiltration 4wk post-surgery in sham and injured adult and aging adult valves. White arrowheads indicate areas of EBD infiltration. **D)** Quantification of EBD intensity shown as a fold change of injured normalized to sham valves. (n=3-6 per group, *:p<0.05, two-tailed unpaired t test).

92

Chapter 4: Concluding Remarks and Clinical Implications

4.1 Valve Growth and Maintenance Transcriptional Profiles

The cardiac valves are dynamic structures that undergo diverse phases of development, remodeling, and maintenance. The embryonic program of valve development has been extensively studied and the valve interstitial cell (VIC) population is known to arise from multiple lineages including endocardial, second heart field, and neural crest, with the addition of epicardial cells for the atrioventricular valves [15, 16]. Immature or developmental VICs are highly proliferative, and thought to be responsible for remodeling the extracellular matrix (ECM) components into stratified layers within the developing valve primordia [17, 18]. After birth, the immature valve continues to develop, however very little is known about this postnatal maturation process. To address this, our study explored the transcriptional changes between the murine postnatal day (PND) 2 developing aortic valve (AoV), and the mature AoV at 4 months of age. Interestingly we note that postnatal remodeling requires a distinct transcriptional program, with the most differentially expressed genes falling into the categories of proliferation, ECM, and immune defense. In contrast to postnatal valves, VICs within the adult mature valve are quiescent and considered homogenous, but emerging data, including that described here in Chapter 2, suggest heterogeneity.

The PND2 valve highly expressed cell cycle promoters and indicators of active proliferation, while the 4 month adult valve showed greater levels of proliferation inhibitors such as *Nox4* and *Sfrp4*, suggesting that proliferation is regulatorily suppressed in the normal adult valve. However, proliferating cells (<1%) were observed in the adult, indicating a possible need for low-level cell turnover and renewal, with the potential for increased activation. In the ECM category, we observed an abundance of various ECM components being produced at both stages, but with distinct expression of certain dominant transcripts. The actively growing PND2 valve more highly expressed proteoglycans *Acan* (*Aggrecan*) and *Vcan* (*Versican*) and fibrillar collagens including *Col9a1* and *Col5a1*, which may provide strength to the valve cusp as it grows. Expression of additional structure stabilizing proteins such as *Frem1/Frem2* and *Nid2* (*Nidogen2*) was also highly increased at this stage. In contrast, the adult valve showed predominant expression of proteoglycans *Dcn* (*Decorin*) and *Bgn* (*Biglycan*) and active transcription of non-fibrillar collagens. These distinct ECM profiles demonstrate the need for a unique ECM composition at different stages, likely due to changing mechanical forces throughout the lifetime of the valve. As RNA-sequencing detects transcripts rather than existing deposited protein, these results further indicate a need for active ECM production in the adult valve, potentially as a renewal mechanism. The adult valve also displayed increased production of defense-related transcripts. While previous studies have clearly demonstrated the existence of an immune cell population in the AoV [30, 34, 35], the role of these cells is still an active area of investigation. This study may contribute insight into the function of these endogenous immune cells and provide the ability to isolate and target specific genes.

Our data provides a window into two stages of the AoV and allows for examination of the transcriptional profiles associated with postnatal growth and active adult maintenance. We have shown that the PND2 AoV profile is strongly oriented towards growth and structural stabilization, while adult valve transcription largely indicates active maintenance through turnover of both cell and ECM components. This assessment is in line with results from other groups demonstrating the ability of valve cells to respond to hemodynamic or signaling changes [22, 27-29, 32, 33]. Although this investigation focused on whole-valve transcription, an additional study from our lab examined transcription of VECs alone at comparable timepoints [60]. Utilizing these two datasets in parallel will provide a platform for inferring endothelial vs interstitial expression and the role and behavior of each cell type at these stages. Further, this study may provide insight into target areas, such as ECM and immune cells, for development of alternative therapeutics to promote growth and active maintenance phenotypes. However, to develop effective therapies it will also be crucial to examine how the active adult maintenance program described here responds in the context of exposure to risk factors for valve disease, including damage or injury.

4.2 Valve Endothelial Damage and Repair

Along with further characterization of the active maintenance observed in the adult AoV, understanding the adaptability and plasticity of the valve will also be essential for treating patients with valve disease. Studies have continued to suggest that endothelial damage or dysfunction is an initiating factor for valve disease development [68-72]. However, few investigations have examined the healthy adult valve response to VEC damage and the associated ability to restore balance and homeostasis. To address this issue, we adapted a non-genetic surgical mouse model of AoV endothelial damage. The procedure was initially designed to produce severe damage to the entire AoV in order to promote disease development [76], while our modifications were designed to produce a more mild endothelial injury which allowed us to examine the possibility for repair in the absence of acute disease. Our results showed that our adapted procedure induced endothelial damage as evidenced by increased permeability of the VEC layer within 6 hours of surgery. However, we observed a return to homeostatic permeability levels within 48 hours of the procedure, indicating that repair had occurred. To our knowledge, this is the first time the adult mammalian valve has been shown to possess native repair capacity.

To further explore the mechanism behind this repair response, we performed bulk RNA-sequencing on sham and injured AoV. Results indicated strong involvement of cell proliferation and the ECM in the injured valve response. With further examination, we confirmed highly increased proliferation of multiple native valve cell types out to 48 hours after injury. Although future work will be necessary to fully appreciate the role and function of each proliferating cell type, it is clear that this is a relevant component of the AoV repair response. Additionally, this data demonstrates that the homeostatic adult valve has the ability to reactivate proliferative programs in response to stimulus, which is encouraging evidence for the development of future therapeutics. RNA-sequencing results implicating the ECM further led us to examine the Tgfβ1-Cthrc1 signaling axis as Cthrc1 is known to be involved in ECM remodeling [163]. We show that Tgfβ1 and Cthrc1 are upregulated after endothelial injury and that this pathway likely promotes proliferation as well as migration of native valve cells in order to repair the VEC barrier. Tgfβ1 signaling has also recently been shown to be involved in the valve regeneration process in zebrafish [100], suggesting a partially conserved mechanism which could be therapeutically targeted. Likewise, Cthrc1 has been implicated in vascular repair [162, 163] and appears to be a promising regulator of wound healing in general [161, 169]. Utilizing our existing *Cthrc1*$^{-/-}$ mouse model in combination with *in vitro* experiments will shed further light on the precise functions of this signaling axis in the repair response, and provide insight into the potential for therapeutic control of valve cell proliferation and migration.

We additionally investigated the capacity for adaptation in aging mice and observe an overall blunted response to damage and an ultimate inability to repair the endothelial barrier. Together with our knowledge about aging and valve disease, this study could partially explain the higher incidence of valve disease in the aging population [147, 182]. While the younger adult valve appears to have the ability to respond to damage and the wear and tear that occurs throughout life, over time the aging adult valve may lose this capacity, leading to an inability to repair and eventual disease development as a result of endothelial damage. This concept is further supported by previous research from our lab showing an overall decline in valve endothelial function with increasing age [60]. Together, these studies imply that the aging valve has a more static biology and is less adaptable, resulting in a decreased ability to respond to changing conditions to prevent disease.

In addition to data insights described here, this study provides a model for future important work investigating the valve injury and repair response as our adaptions to create a milder level of injury allows for examination of factors which may be lost in a severe disease model. Although our results have focused on the short-term damage response, longer-term timepoints will also be needed to fully understand the AoV adaption to stimulation and injury. Additionally, many variations on the model could be utilized to examine different aspects of valve injury and disease. For example, producing a mild injury by repeating the procedure multiple times in a single animal may more accurately mimic low-level physiological wear and tear. This model could also be used in combination with transgenic models of valve disease to examine the interaction between genetic and physical factors in disease development.

Our results together demonstrate that the adult valve, traditionally thought to be quiescent and inactive, has the ability to adapt and activate specific programs when stimulated or damaged. In combination with the study described in Chapter 2, this data shifts our understanding of the homeostatic adult valve and demonstrates a more active and responsive valve biology. This perspective will be critical for understanding valve disease pathology as well as developing targeted therapeutics. We anticipate that this first examination of the mammalian adult valve damage response will motivate future work and contribute valuable insight regarding the dynamic nature of the adult AoV and the potential for both endogenous and therapeutic repair to prevent or slow valve disease progression.

4.3 Clinical Implications

Left untreated, valve disease can lead to heart failure and eventually death [3]. However, despite the increasing prevalence, surgical repair or replacement remains the only effective treatment. Although techniques have improved and surgery is generally well-tolerated, risks still exist and some patients with existing comorbidities are not candidates for surgery [79, 80]. Additionally, the most widely used replacement valve materials have their own disadvantages. Tissue valves are not particularly durable and often involve repeat replacement surgery, while mechanical valves increase the risk of thrombus and require the continual use of anticoagulation drugs [88, 89]. Due to these potential complications, a non-surgical therapeutic treatment for valve disease would be advantageous and considerably improve patient quality of life. Some attempts have been made to utilize existing pharmaceuticals, such as statins and beta-blockers, to treat valve disease. However, clinical results have been inconsistent and outcomes from these treatments alone are not extremely promising [15, 81-84, 183, 184].

As discussed, a deep understanding of valvular biology is essential for discovering methods to combat valve disease development and to treat existing disease. Here, our results provide a foundation for understanding the dynamic nature of adult valve homeostasis and response to stimulus. Our large transcriptomic data sets can be utilized to identify potential therapeutic targets, two of which (Tgfβ1 and Cthrc1) we examined more thoroughly in this study. Additionally, our modified model of valve endothelial injury can be utilized in future investigations to evaluate the injury response in different contexts, as well as to test the success of potential therapeutic repair methods. The data described here also provides valuable insight into clinical intervention at different points in development. Our results show that different types of therapies may be necessary to completely harness the endogenous mechanisms in place at each stage. For example, treating an infant with congenital valve disease will likely require regulation and control of different pathways than treating an adult with acquired valve disease. Our RNA-sequencing data comparing growth and maintenance profiles provides a starting point to understand these nuances. Additionally, our study implies that the damage response and repair capacity likely shifts throughout life. Although we examined adults and aging adults, the trends we observed may indicate that younger valves have an even greater ability to repair after damage. Patients with congenital valve disease also exhibit valve endothelial damage and dysfunction [68, 185, 186], and our studies here may suggest that these very young valves are more amenable to upregulation of repair pathways or endogenous repair. However, as evidenced by differences in regenerative ability between zebrafish and mammals, future work studying the valve repair response in various species at different ages, including humans, will be required.

In closing, our data has contributed a therapeutically relevant basis for understanding valvular biology in growth and maintenance stages. Particularly, we have provided insight into the active and adaptable adult valve which we show, for the first time, has the innate ability to self-repair in response to endothelial damage. Going forward, we expect that the maintenance and repair mechanisms highlighted here can be therapeutically harnessed to promote a healthy valve structure despite the presence of risk factors.

References

1. Schoen, F.J., *Mechanisms of function and disease of natural and replacement heart valves.* Annu Rev Pathol, 2012. **7**: p. 161-83.
2. Hinton, R.B., Jr., et al., *Extracellular matrix remodeling and organization in developing and diseased aortic valves.* Circ Res, 2006. **98**(11): p. 1431-8.
3. Hinton, R.B. and K.E. Yutzey, *Heart valve structure and function in development and disease.* Annu Rev Physiol, 2011. **73**: p. 29-46.
4. Misfeld, M. and H.H. Sievers, *Heart valve macro- and microstructure.* Philos Trans R Soc Lond B Biol Sci, 2007. **362**(1484): p. 1421-36.
5. Sacks, M.S., W. David Merryman, and D.E. Schmidt, *On the biomechanics of heart valve function.* J Biomech, 2009. **42**(12): p. 1804-24.
6. MacGrogan, D., et al., *How to make a heart valve: from embryonic development to bioengineering of living valve substitutes.* Cold Spring Harb Perspect Med, 2014. **4**(11): p. a013912.
7. Balachandran, K., P. Sucosky, and A.P. Yoganathan, *Hemodynamics and mechanobiology of aortic valve inflammation and calcification.* Int J Inflam, 2011. **2011**: p. 263870.
8. Arjunon, S., et al., *Aortic valve: mechanical environment and mechanobiology.* Ann Biomed Eng, 2013. **41**(7): p. 1331-46.
9. Mongkoldhumrongkul, N., et al., *Effect of Side-Specific Valvular Shear Stress on the Content of Extracellular Matrix in Aortic Valves.* Cardiovasc Eng Technol, 2018. **9**(2): p. 151-157.
10. Bader, A., et al., *Tissue engineering of heart valves--human endothelial cell seeding of detergent acellularized porcine valves.* Eur J Cardiothorac Surg, 1998. **14**(3): p. 279-84.
11. Exposito, J.Y., et al., *The fibrillar collagen family.* Int J Mol Sci, 2010. **11**(2): p. 407-26.
12. Lehmann, S., et al., *Mechanical strain and the aortic valve: influence on fibroblasts, extracellular matrix, and potential stenosis.* Ann Thorac Surg, 2009. **88**(5): p. 1476-83.
13. Vesely, I., *The role of elastin in aortic valve mechanics.* J Biomech, 1998. **31**(2): p. 115-23.
14. Chen, J.H. and C.A. Simmons, *Cell-matrix interactions in the pathobiology of calcific aortic valve disease: critical roles for matricellular, matricrine, and matrix mechanics cues.* Circ Res, 2011. **108**(12): p. 1510-24.

15.   Dutta, P., et al., *Genetic and Developmental Contributors to Aortic Stenosis.* Circ Res, 2021 (In Press).

16.   Wu, B., et al., *Developmental Mechanisms of Aortic Valve Malformation and Disease.* Annu Rev Physiol, 2017. **79**: p. 21-41.

17.   Liu, A.C., V.R. Joag, and A.I. Gotlieb, *The emerging role of valve interstitial cell phenotypes in regulating heart valve pathobiology.* Am J Pathol, 2007. **171**(5): p. 1407-18.

18.   Taylor, P.M., et al., *The cardiac valve interstitial cell.* Int J Biochem Cell Biol, 2003. **35**(2): p. 113-8.

19.   Duan, B., et al., *Active tissue stiffness modulation controls valve interstitial cell phenotype and osteogenic potential in 3D culture.* Acta Biomater, 2016. **36**: p. 42-54.

20.   Latif, N., et al., *Characterization of molecules mediating cell-cell communication in human cardiac valve interstitial cells.* Cell Biochem Biophys, 2006. **45**(3): p. 255-64.

21.   Latif, N., et al., *Molecules mediating cell-ECM and cell-cell communication in human heart valves.* Cell Biochem Biophys, 2005. **43**(2): p. 275-87.

22.   Mongkoldhumrongkul, N., M.H. Yacoub, and A.H. Chester, *Valve Endothelial Cells - Not Just Any Old Endothelial Cells.* Curr Vasc Pharmacol, 2016. **14**(2): p. 146-54.

23.   El-Hamamsy, I., et al., *Endothelium-dependent regulation of the mechanical properties of aortic valve cusps.* J Am Coll Cardiol, 2009. **53**(16): p. 1448-55.

24.   Armstrong, E.J. and J. Bischoff, *Heart valve development: endothelial cell signaling and differentiation.* Circ Res, 2004. **95**(5): p. 459-70.

25.   Huk, D.J., et al., *Valve Endothelial Cell-Derived Tgfbeta1 Signaling Promotes Nuclear Localization of Sox9 in Interstitial Cells Associated With Attenuated Calcification.* Arterioscler Thromb Vasc Biol, 2016. **36**(2): p. 328-38.

26.   Bosse, K., et al., *Endothelial nitric oxide signaling regulates Notch1 in aortic valve disease.* J Mol Cell Cardiol, 2013. **60**: p. 27-35.

27.   Leopold, J.A., *Cellular mechanisms of aortic valve calcification.* Circ Cardiovasc Interv, 2012. **5**(4): p. 605-14.

28.   Butcher, J.T. and R.M. Nerem, *Valvular endothelial cells and the mechanoregulation of valvular pathology.* Philos Trans R Soc Lond B Biol Sci, 2007. **362**(1484): p. 1445-57.

29.   Chester, A.H., et al., *The living aortic valve: From molecules to function.* Glob Cardiol Sci Pract, 2014. **2014**(1): p. 52-77.

30.   Hulin, A., et al., *Maturation of heart valve cell populations during postnatal remodeling.* Development, 2019. **146**(12).

31.   Simmons, C.A., et al., *Spatial heterogeneity of endothelial phenotypes correlates with side-specific vulnerability to calcification in normal porcine aortic valves.* Circ Res, 2005. **96**(7): p. 792-9.

32.   Butcher, J.T., et al., *Unique morphology and focal adhesion development of valvular endothelial cells in static and fluid flow environments.* Arterioscler Thromb Vasc Biol, 2004. **24**(8): p. 1429-34.

33.   Gould, S.T., et al., *The role of valvular endothelial cell paracrine signaling and matrix elasticity on valvular interstitial cell activation.* Biomaterials, 2014. **35**(11): p. 3596-606.

34.   Hulin, A., et al., *Macrophage Transitions in Heart Valve Development and Myxomatous Valve Disease.* Arterioscler Thromb Vasc Biol, 2018. **38**(3): p. 636-644.

35.   Hajdu, Z., et al., *Recruitment of bone marrow-derived valve interstitial cells is a normal homeostatic process.* J Mol Cell Cardiol, 2011. **51**(6): p. 955-65.

36.   Anstine, L.J., et al., *Contribution of Extra-Cardiac Cells in Murine Heart Valves is Age-Dependent.* J Am Heart Assoc, 2017. **6**(10).

37.   Sanchez-Pina, J., et al., *Pigmentation of the aortic and pulmonary valves in C57BL/6J x Balb/cByJ hybrid mice of different coat colours.* Anat Histol Embryol, 2019. **48**(5): p. 429-436.

38.   Hong, Y., et al., *Melanocytes and Skin Immunity.* J Investig Dermatol Symp Proc, 2015. **17**(1): p. 37-9.

39.   Balani, K., et al., *Melanocyte pigmentation stiffens murine cardiac tricuspid valve leaflet.* J R Soc Interface, 2009. **6**(40): p. 1097-102.

40.   Carneiro, F., et al., *Relationships between melanocytes, mechanical properties and extracellular matrix composition in mouse heart valves.* J Long Term Eff Med Implants, 2015. **25**(1-2): p. 17-26.

41.   Martin, P.S., et al., *Embryonic Development of the Bicuspid Aortic Valve.* J Cardiovasc Dev Dis, 2015. **2**(4): p. 248-272.

42.   Lopez-Sanchez, C. and V. Garcia-Martinez, *Molecular determinants of cardiac specification.* Cardiovasc Res, 2011. **91**(2): p. 185-95.

43.   Henderson, D.J., L. Eley, and B. Chaudhry, *New Concepts in the Development and Malformation of the Arterial Valves.* J Cardiovasc Dev Dis, 2020. **7**(4).

44.   Lin, C.J., et al., *Partitioning the heart: mechanisms of cardiac septation and valve development.* Development, 2012. **139**(18): p. 3277-99.

45.   Combs, M.D. and K.E. Yutzey, *Heart valve development: regulatory networks in development and disease.* Circ Res, 2009. **105**(5): p. 408-21.

46.   Menon, V. and J. Lincoln, *The Genetic Regulation of Aortic Valve Development and Calcific Disease.* Front Cardiovasc Med, 2018. **5**: p. 162.

47.   Gomez Stallons, M.V., et al., *Molecular Mechanisms of Heart Valve Development and Disease*, in *Etiology and Morphogenesis of Congenital Heart Disease: From Gene Function and Cellular Interaction to Morphology*, T. Nakanishi, et al., Editors. 2016: Tokyo. p. 145-151.

48.   Bischoff, J. and E. Aikawa, *Progenitor cells confer plasticity to cardiac valve endothelium.* J Cardiovasc Transl Res, 2011. **4**(6): p. 710-9.

49.   Bischoff, J., *Endothelial-to-Mesenchymal Transition.* Circ Res, 2019. **124**(8): p. 1163-1165.

50.   Jiang, X., et al., *Fate of the mammalian cardiac neural crest.* Development, 2000. **127**(8): p. 1607-16.

51.   Jiang, X., et al., *Normal fate and altered function of the cardiac neural crest cell lineage in retinoic acid receptor mutant embryos.* Mech Dev, 2002. **117**(1-2): p. 115-22.

52.   Verzi, M.P., et al., *The right ventricle, outflow tract, and ventricular septum comprise a restricted expression domain within the secondary/anterior heart field.* Dev Biol, 2005. **287**(1): p. 134-45.

53.   Lincoln, J., C.M. Alfieri, and K.E. Yutzey, *Development of heart valve leaflets and supporting apparatus in chicken and mouse embryos.* Dev Dyn, 2004. **230**(2): p. 239-50.

54.   de Lange, F.J., et al., *Lineage and morphogenetic analysis of the cardiac valves.* Circ Res, 2004. **95**(6): p. 645-54.

55.   Mifflin, J.J., et al., *Intercalated cushion cells within the cardiac outflow tract are derived from the myocardial troponin T type 2 (Tnnt2) Cre lineage.* Dev Dyn, 2018. **247**(8): p. 1005-1017.

56.   Leung, C., et al., *Rac1 Signaling Is Required for Anterior Second Heart Field Cellular Organization and Cardiac Outflow Tract Development.* J Am Heart Assoc, 2015. **5**(1).

57.   Aikawa, E., et al., *Human semilunar cardiac valve remodeling by activated cells from fetus to adult: implications for postnatal adaptation, pathology, and tissue engineering.* Circulation, 2006. **113**(10): p. 1344-52.

58.   Dutta, P. and J. Lincoln, *Calcific Aortic Valve Disease: a Developmental Biology Perspective.* Curr Cardiol Rep, 2018. **20**(4): p. 21.

59.   Wirrig, E.E. and K.E. Yutzey, *Transcriptional regulation of heart valve development and disease.* Cardiovasc Pathol, 2011. **20**(3): p. 162-7.

60.   Anstine, L.J., et al., *Growth and maturation of heart valves leads to changes in endothelial cell distribution, impaired function, decreased metabolism and reduced cell proliferation.* J Mol Cell Cardiol, 2016. **100**: p. 72-82.

61.   Supino, P.G., et al., *The epidemiology of valvular heart disease: a growing public health problem.* Heart Fail Clin, 2006. **2**(4): p. 379-93.

62.   Nkomo, V.T., et al., *Burden of valvular heart diseases: a population-based study.* Lancet, 2006. **368**(9540): p. 1005-11.

63.   Chen, H.Y., J.C. Engert, and G. Thanassoulis, *Risk factors for valvular calcification.* Curr Opin Endocrinol Diabetes Obes, 2019. **26**(2): p. 96-102.

64.   Cho, K.I., et al., *Inflammatory and metabolic mechanisms underlying the calcific aortic valve disease.* Atherosclerosis, 2018. **277**: p. 60-65.

65.   Eveborn, G.W., et al., *The evolving epidemiology of valvular aortic stenosis. the Tromso study.* Heart, 2013. **99**(6): p. 396-400.

66.   Balaoing, L.R., et al., *Age-related changes in aortic valve hemostatic protein regulation.* Arterioscler Thromb Vasc Biol, 2014. **34**(1): p. 72-80.

67.   Gumpangseth, T., P. Mahakkanukrauh, and S. Das, *Gross age-related changes and diseases in human heart valves.* Anat Cell Biol, 2019. **52**(1): p. 25-33.

68.	Kostyunin, A.E., et al., *Development of calcific aortic valve disease: Do we know enough for new clinical trials?* J Mol Cell Cardiol, 2019. **132**: p. 189-209.

69.	Li, C., S. Xu, and A.I. Gotlieb, *The progression of calcific aortic valve disease through injury, cell dysfunction, and disruptive biologic and physical force feedback loops.* Cardiovasc Pathol, 2013. **22**(1): p. 1-8.

70.	Leask, R.L., N. Jain, and J. Butany, *Endothelium and valvular diseases of the heart.* Microsc Res Tech, 2003. **60**(2): p. 129-37.

71.	Poggianti, E., et al., *Aortic valve sclerosis is associated with systemic endothelial dysfunction.* J Am Coll Cardiol, 2003. **41**(1): p. 136-41.

72.	Tao, G., J.D. Kotick, and J. Lincoln, *Heart valve development, maintenance, and disease: the role of endothelial cells.* Curr Top Dev Biol, 2012. **100**: p. 203-32.

73.	Mohler, E.R., 3rd, *Mechanisms of aortic valve calcification.* Am J Cardiol, 2004. **94**(11): p. 1396-402, A6.

74.	Otto, C.M., et al., *Characterization of the early lesion of 'degenerative' valvular aortic stenosis. Histological and immunohistochemical studies.* Circulation, 1994. **90**(2): p. 844-53.

75.	Lee, Y.S. and Y.Y. Chou, *Endothelial alterations and senile calcific aortic stenosis: an electron microscopic observation.* Proc Natl Sci Counc Repub China B, 1997. **21**(4): p. 137-43.

76.	Honda, S., et al., *A novel mouse model of aortic valve stenosis induced by direct wire injury.* Arterioscler Thromb Vasc Biol, 2014. **34**(2): p. 270-8.

77.	Hjortnaes, J., et al., *Valvular interstitial cells suppress calcification of valvular endothelial cells.* Atherosclerosis, 2015. **242**(1): p. 251-260.

78.	Yadgir, S., et al., *Global, Regional, and National Burden of Calcific Aortic Valve and Degenerative Mitral Valve Diseases, 1990-2017.* Circulation, 2020. **141**(21): p. 1670-1680.

79.	Baumgartner, H., *The 2017 ESC/EACTS guidelines on the management of valvular heart disease : What is new and what has changed compared to the 2012 guidelines?* Wien Klin Wochenschr, 2018. **130**(5-6): p. 168-171.

80.	Kanwar, A., J.J. Thaden, and V.T. Nkomo, *Management of Patients With Aortic Valve Stenosis.* Mayo Clin Proc, 2018. **93**(4): p. 488-508.

81.	Antonini-Canterin, F., et al., *Stage-related effect of statin treatment on the progression of aortic valve sclerosis and stenosis.* Am J Cardiol, 2008. **102**(6): p. 738-42.

82.	Bellamy, M.F., et al., *Association of cholesterol levels, hydroxymethylglutaryl coenzyme-A reductase inhibitor treatment, and progression of aortic stenosis in the community.* J Am Coll Cardiol, 2002. **40**(10): p. 1723-30.

83.	Dichtl, W., et al., *Prognosis and risk factors in patients with asymptomatic aortic stenosis and their modulation by atorvastatin (20 mg).* Am J Cardiol, 2008. **102**(6): p. 743-8.

84.	Cowell, S.J., et al., *A randomized trial of intensive lipid-lowering therapy in calcific aortic stenosis.* N Engl J Med, 2005. **352**(23): p. 2389-97.

85.   Dawkins, S. and R.R. Makkar, *Balloon Aortic Valvuloplasty: Is It Still Relevant?* Circ Cardiovasc Interv, 2017. **10**(5).

86.   Sandhu, K., et al., *Balloon aortic valvuloplasty in contemporary practice.* J Interv Cardiol, 2017. **30**(3): p. 212-216.

87.   Nwaejike, N., et al., *Balloon aortic valvuloplasty as a bridge to aortic valve surgery for severe aortic stenosis.* Interact Cardiovasc Thorac Surg, 2015. **20**(3): p. 429-35.

88.   Baldwin, A.C.W. and G. Tolis, Jr., *Tissue Valve Degeneration and Mechanical Valve Failure.* Curr Treat Options Cardiovasc Med, 2019. **21**(7): p. 33.

89.   Koziarz, A., et al., *Modes of bioprosthetic valve failure: a narrative review.* Curr Opin Cardiol, 2020. **35**(2): p. 123-132.

90.   Foglia, M.J. and K.D. Poss, *Building and re-building the heart by cardiomyocyte proliferation.* Development, 2016. **143**(5): p. 729-40.

91.   Vujic, A., N. Natarajan, and R.T. Lee, *Molecular mechanisms of heart regeneration.* Semin Cell Dev Biol, 2020. **100**: p. 20-28.

92.   Senyo, S.E., R.T. Lee, and B. Kuhn, *Cardiac regeneration based on mechanisms of cardiomyocyte proliferation and differentiation.* Stem Cell Res, 2014. **13**(3 Pt B): p. 532-41.

93.   Bassat, E., et al., *The extracellular matrix protein agrin promotes heart regeneration in mice.* Nature, 2017. **547**(7662): p. 179-184.

94.   Tzahor, E. and K.D. Poss, *Cardiac regeneration strategies: Staying young at heart.* Science, 2017. **356**(6342): p. 1035-1039.

95.   Cardoso, A.C., A.H.M. Pereira, and H.A. Sadek, *Mechanisms of Neonatal Heart Regeneration.* Curr Cardiol Rep, 2020. **22**(5): p. 33.

96.   Pronobis, M.I. and K.D. Poss, *Signals for cardiomyocyte proliferation during zebrafish heart regeneration.* Curr Opin Physiol, 2020. **14**: p. 78-85.

97.   Gonzalez-Rosa, J.M., C.E. Burns, and C.G. Burns, *Zebrafish heart regeneration: 15 years of discoveries.* Regeneration (Oxf), 2017. **4**(3): p. 105-123.

98.   McDonald, A.I., et al., *Endothelial Regeneration of Large Vessels Is a Biphasic Process Driven by Local Cells with Distinct Proliferative Capacities.* Cell Stem Cell, 2018. **23**(2): p. 210-225 e6.

99.   Kefalos, P., et al., *Reactivation of Notch signaling is required for cardiac valve regeneration.* Sci Rep, 2019. **9**(1): p. 16059.

100.   Bensimon-Brito, A., et al., *TGF-beta Signaling Promotes Tissue Formation during Cardiac Valve Regeneration in Adult Zebrafish.* Dev Cell, 2020. **52**(1): p. 9-20 e7.

101.   Lester, W.M. and A.I. Gotlieb, *In vitro repair of the wounded porcine mitral valve.* Circ Res, 1988. **62**(4): p. 833-45.

102.   Horne, T.E., et al., *Dynamic Heterogeneity of the Heart Valve Interstitial Cell Population in Mitral Valve Health and Disease.* J Cardiovasc Dev Dis, 2015. **2**(3): p. 214-232.

103.   Lincoln, J. and K.E. Yutzey, *Molecular and developmental mechanisms of congenital heart valve disease.* Birth Defects Res A Clin Mol Teratol, 2011. **91**(6): p. 526-34.

104.   Benjamin, E.J., et al., *Heart Disease and Stroke Statistics-2017 Update: A Report From the American Heart Association.* Circulation, 2017. **135**(10): p. e146-e603.

105.   Bach, D.S., et al., *Prevalence, referral patterns, testing, and surgery in aortic valve disease: leaving women and elderly patients behind?* J Heart Valve Dis, 2007. **16**(4): p. 362-9.

106.   Etnel, J.R., et al., *Outcome after aortic valve replacement in children: A systematic review and meta-analysis.* J Thorac Cardiovasc Surg, 2016. **151**(1): p. 143-52 e1-3.

107.   Porrello, E.R., et al., *Transient regenerative potential of the neonatal mouse heart.* Science, 2011. **331**(6020): p. 1078-80.

108.   Soonpaa, M.H. and L.J. Field, *Assessment of cardiomyocyte DNA synthesis in normal and injured adult mouse hearts.* Am J Physiol, 1997. **272**(1 Pt 2): p. H220-6.

109.   Li, F., et al., *Rapid transition of cardiac myocytes from hyperplasia to hypertrophy during postnatal development.* J Mol Cell Cardiol, 1996. **28**(8): p. 1737-46.

110.   Heallen, T., et al., *Hippo pathway inhibits Wnt signaling to restrain cardiomyocyte proliferation and heart size.* Science, 2011. **332**(6028): p. 458-61.

111.   Xin, M., et al., *Hippo pathway effector Yap promotes cardiac regeneration.* Proc Natl Acad Sci U S A, 2013. **110**(34): p. 13839-44.

112.   Peacock, J.D., et al., *Temporal and spatial expression of collagens during murine atrioventricular heart valve development and maintenance.* Dev Dyn, 2008. **237**(10): p. 3051-8.

113.   de Hoon, M.J., et al., *Open source clustering software.* Bioinformatics, 2004. **20**(9): p. 1453-4.

114.   Huang da, W., B.T. Sherman, and R.A. Lempicki, *Systematic and integrative analysis of large gene lists using DAVID bioinformatics resources.* Nat Protoc, 2009. **4**(1): p. 44-57.

115.   Walter, W., F. Sanchez-Cabo, and M. Ricote, *GOplot: an R package for visually combining expression data with functional analysis.* Bioinformatics, 2015. **31**(17): p. 2912-4.

116.   Huk, D.J., et al., *Increased dietary intake of vitamin A promotes aortic valve calcification in vivo.* Arterioscler Thromb Vasc Biol, 2013. **33**(2): p. 285-93.

117.   Jurikova, M., et al., *Ki67, PCNA, and MCM proteins: Markers of proliferation in the diagnosis of breast cancer.* Acta Histochem, 2016. **118**(5): p. 544-52.

118.   Wadugu, B. and B. Kuhn, *The role of neuregulin/ErbB2/ErbB4 signaling in the heart with special focus on effects on cardiomyocyte proliferation.* Am J Physiol Heart Circ Physiol, 2012. **302**(11): p. H2139-47.

119. Kalwa, H. and T. Michel, *The MARCKS protein plays a critical role in phosphatidylinositol 4,5-bisphosphate metabolism and directed cell movement in vascular endothelial cells.* J Biol Chem, 2011. **286**(3): p. 2320-30.

120. Chien, A.J., W.H. Conrad, and R.T. Moon, *A Wnt survival guide: from flies to human disease.* J Invest Dermatol, 2009. **129**(7): p. 1614-27.

121. Jung, J.J., et al., *Multimodality and molecular imaging of matrix metalloproteinase activation in calcific aortic valve disease.* J Nucl Med, 2015. **56**(6): p. 933-8.

122. Perrotta, I., et al., *Matrix Metalloproteinase-9 Expression in Calcified Human Aortic Valves: A Histopathologic, Immunohistochemical, and Ultrastructural Study.* Appl Immunohistochem Mol Morphol, 2016. **24**(2): p. 128-37.

123. Moesgaard, S.G., et al., *Matrix metalloproteinases (MMPs), tissue inhibitors of metalloproteinases (TIMPs) and transforming growth factor-beta (TGF-beta) in advanced canine myxomatous mitral valve disease.* Res Vet Sci, 2014. **97**(3): p. 560-7.

124. Ye, S., et al., *Progression of coronary atherosclerosis is associated with a common genetic variant of the human stromelysin-1 promoter which results in reduced gene expression.* J Biol Chem, 1996. **271**(22): p. 13055-60.

125. Banik, D., et al., *MMP3-mediated tumor progression is controlled transcriptionally by a novel IRF8-MMP3 interaction.* Oncotarget, 2015. **6**(17): p. 15164-79.

126. Mehner, C., et al., *Tumor cell expression of MMP3 as a prognostic factor for poor survival in pancreatic, pulmonary, and mammary carcinoma.* Genes Cancer, 2015. **6**(11-12): p. 480-9.

127. Narumiya, S., Y. Sugimoto, and F. Ushikubi, *Prostanoid receptors: structures, properties, and functions.* Physiol Rev, 1999. **79**(4): p. 1193-226.

128. Wirrig, E.E., et al., *COX2 inhibition reduces aortic valve calcification in vivo.* Arterioscler Thromb Vasc Biol, 2015. **35**(4): p. 938-47.

129. Kunimoto, H., et al., *Chemerin promotes the proliferation and migration of vascular smooth muscle and increases mouse blood pressure.* Am J Physiol Heart Circ Physiol, 2015. **309**(5): p. H1017-28.

130. Chu, Y., et al., *Fibrotic Aortic Valve Stenosis in Hypercholesterolemic/Hypertensive Mice.* Arterioscler Thromb Vasc Biol, 2016. **36**(3): p. 466-74.

131. Ouyang, B., et al., *Human Bub1: a putative spindle checkpoint kinase closely linked to cell proliferation.* Cell Growth Differ, 1998. **9**(10): p. 877-85.

132. Kalin, T.V., V. Ustiyan, and V.V. Kalinichenko, *Multiple faces of FoxM1 transcription factor: lessons from transgenic mouse models.* Cell Cycle, 2011. **10**(3): p. 396-405.

133. Schroder, K., et al., *Nox4 acts as a switch between differentiation and proliferation in preadipocytes.* Arterioscler Thromb Vasc Biol, 2009. **29**(2): p. 239-45.

134.	Meloche, S. and J. Pouyssegur, *The ERK1/2 mitogen-activated protein kinase pathway as a master regulator of the G1- to S-phase transition.* Oncogene, 2007. **26**(22): p. 3227-39.

135.	Maganga, R., et al., *Secreted Frizzled related protein-4 (sFRP4) promotes epidermal differentiation and apoptosis.* Biochem Biophys Res Commun, 2008. **377**(2): p. 606-611.

136.	Perumal, V., et al., *Therapeutic approach to target mesothelioma cancer cells using the Wnt antagonist, secreted frizzled-related protein 4: Metabolic state of cancer cells.* Exp Cell Res, 2016. **341**(2): p. 218-24.

137.	Cole-Jeffrey, C.T., et al., *Progressive anatomical closure of foramen ovale in normal neonatal mouse hearts.* Anat Rec (Hoboken), 2012. **295**(5): p. 764-8.

138.	Steed, E., F. Boselli, and J. Vermot, *Hemodynamics driven cardiac valve morphogenesis.* Biochim Biophys Acta, 2016. **1863**(7 Pt B): p. 1760-6.

139.	Pavlakis, E., R. Chiotaki, and G. Chalepakis, *The role of Fras1/Frem proteins in the structure and function of basement membrane.* Int J Biochem Cell Biol, 2011. **43**(4): p. 487-95.

140.	Kohfeldt, E., et al., *Nidogen-2: a new basement membrane protein with diverse binding properties.* J Mol Biol, 1998. **282**(1): p. 99-109.

141.	Yutzey, K.E., *Cardiomyocyte Proliferation: Teaching an Old Dogma New Tricks.* Circ Res, 2017. **120**(4): p. 627-629.

142.	Schoen, F.J., *Evolving concepts of cardiac valve dynamics: the continuum of development, functional structure, pathobiology, and tissue engineering.* Circulation, 2008. **118**(18): p. 1864-80.

143.	Erhart-Hledik, J.C., et al., *A relationship between mechanically-induced changes in serum cartilage oligomeric matrix protein (COMP) and changes in cartilage thickness after 5 years.* Osteoarthritis Cartilage, 2012. **20**(11): p. 1309-15.

144.	Batista, M.A., et al., *Nanomechanical phenotype of chondroadherin-null murine articular cartilage.* Matrix Biol, 2014. **38**: p. 84-90.

145.	Stephens, E.H., C.K. Chu, and K.J. Grande-Allen, *Valve proteoglycan content and glycosaminoglycan fine structure are unique to microstructure, mechanical load and age: Relevance to an age-specific tissue-engineered heart valve.* Acta Biomater, 2008. **4**(5): p. 1148-60.

146.	Li, C., S. Xu, and A.I. Gotlieb, *The response to valve injury. A paradigm to understand the pathogenesis of heart valve disease.* Cardiovasc Pathol, 2011. **20**(3): p. 183-90.

147.	Coffey, S., B.J. Cairns, and B. Iung, *The modern epidemiology of heart valve disease.* Heart, 2016. **102**(1): p. 75-85.

148.	Gomez-Stallons, M.V., et al., *Calcification and extracellular matrix dysregulation in human postmortem and surgical aortic valves.* Heart, 2019. **105**(21): p. 1616-1621.

149.	O'Donnell, A. and K.E. Yutzey, *Mechanisms of heart valve development and disease.* Development, 2020. **147**(13).

150.   Riddle, J.M., D.J. Magilligan, Jr., and P.D. Stein, *Surface topography of stenotic aortic valves by scanning electron microscopy.* Circulation, 1980. **61**(3): p. 496-502.

151.   Isner, J.M., *Acute catastrophic complications of balloon aortic valvuloplasty. The Mansfield Scientific Aortic Valvuloplasty Registry Investigators.* J Am Coll Cardiol, 1991. **17**(6): p. 1436-44.

152.   Wang, A., J.K. Harrison, and T.M. Bashore, *Balloon aortic valvuloplasty.* Prog Cardiovasc Dis, 1997. **40**(1): p. 27-36.

153.   Zampetaki, A., J.P. Kirton, and Q. Xu, *Vascular repair by endothelial progenitor cells.* Cardiovasc Res, 2008. **78**(3): p. 413-21.

154.   Lester, W.M., et al., *Bovine mitral valve organ culture: role of interstitial cells in repair of valvular injury.* J Mol Cell Cardiol, 1992. **24**(1): p. 43-53.

155.   Schneider, C.A., W.S. Rasband, and K.W. Eliceiri, *NIH Image to ImageJ: 25 years of image analysis.* Nat Methods, 2012. **9**(7): p. 671-5.

156.   Benjamini, Y. and Y. Hochberg, *Controlling the False Discovery Rate: A Practical and Powerful Approach to Multiple Testing.* J R Stat Soc B, 1995. **57**: p. 289-300.

157.   Sharov, A., D. Dudekula, and M. KO, *Principal component and significance analysis of microarrays with NIA Array Analysis tool. Bioinformatics.* Bioinformatics, 2005. **21**.

158.   De Hoon, M., et al., *Open Source Clustering Software.* . Bioinformatics, 2004. **20**.

159.   Huang da, W., B.T. Sherman, and R.A. Lempicki, *Bioinformatics enrichment tools: paths toward the comprehensive functional analysis of large gene lists.* Nucleic Acids Res, 2009. **37**(1): p. 1-13.

160.   Lawlor, D.P. and M.L. Horton, 3rd, *Nonmalignant loculated ascites.* Am J Gastroenterol, 1989. **84**(12): p. 1583-4.

161.   Qin, S., et al., *CTHRC1 promotes wound repair by increasing M2 macrophages via regulating the TGF-beta and notch pathways.* Biomed Pharmacother, 2019. **113**: p. 108594.

162.   LeClair, R.J., et al., *Cthrc1 is a novel inhibitor of transforming growth factor-beta signaling and neointimal lesion formation.* Circ Res, 2007. **100**(6): p. 826-33.

163.   Pyagay, P., et al., *Collagen triple helix repeat containing 1, a novel secreted protein in injured and diseased arteries, inhibits collagen expression and promotes cell migration.* Circ Res, 2005. **96**(2): p. 261-8.

164.   Durmus, T., et al., *Expression analysis of the novel gene collagen triple helix repeat containing-1 (Cthrc1).* Gene Expr Patterns, 2006. **6**(8): p. 935-40.

165.   Mei, D., et al., *The Role of CTHRC1 in Regulation of Multiple Signaling and Tumor Progression and Metastasis.* Mediators Inflamm, 2020. **2020**: p. 9578701.

166.   Ganguly, S.S., et al., *Loss of Myeloid-Specific TGF-beta Signaling Decreases CTHRC1 to Downregulate bFGF and the Development of H1993-Induced Osteolytic Bone Lesions.* Cancers (Basel), 2018. **10**(12).

167. Wang, P., et al., *CTHRC1 is upregulated by promoter demethylation and transforming growth factor-beta1 and may be associated with metastasis in human gastric cancer.* Cancer Sci, 2012. **103**(7): p. 1327-33.

168. Lv, Y., et al., *CTHRC1 overexpression promotes ectopic endometrial stromal cell proliferation, migration and invasion via activation of the Wnt/beta-catenin pathway.* Reprod Biomed Online, 2020. **40**(1): p. 26-32.

169. Ruiz-Villalba, A., et al., *Single-Cell RNA Sequencing Analysis Reveals a Crucial Role for CTHRC1 (Collagen Triple Helix Repeat Containing 1) Cardiac Fibroblasts After Myocardial Infarction.* Circulation, 2020. **142**(19): p. 1831-1847.

170. Molin, D.G., et al., *Expression patterns of Tgfbeta1-3 associate with myocardialisation of the outflow tract and the development of the epicardium and the fibrous heart skeleton.* Dev Dyn, 2003. **227**(3): p. 431-44.

171. Barnette, D.N., et al., *Tgfbeta-Smad and MAPK signaling mediate scleraxis and proteoglycan expression in heart valves.* J Mol Cell Cardiol, 2013. **65**: p. 137-46.

172. Wang, C., et al., *High expression of Collagen Triple Helix Repeat Containing 1 (CTHRC1) facilitates progression of oesophageal squamous cell carcinoma through MAPK/MEK/ERK/FRA-1 activation.* J Exp Clin Cancer Res, 2017. **36**(1): p. 84.

173. Ota, I., et al., *Induction of a MT1-MMP and MT2-MMP-dependent basement membrane transmigration program in cancer cells by Snail1.* Proc Natl Acad Sci U S A, 2009. **106**(48): p. 20318-23.

174. Jiang, W., et al., *CD44 regulates pancreatic cancer invasion through MT1-MMP.* Mol Cancer Res, 2015. **13**(1): p. 9-15.

175. Kim, A.J., et al., *Deficiency of Circulating Monocytes Ameliorates the Progression of Myxomatous Valve Degeneration in Marfan Syndrome.* Circulation, 2020. **141**(2): p. 132-146.

176. Kim, A.J., N. Xu, and K.E. Yutzey, *Macrophage lineages in heart valve development and disease.* Cardiovasc Res, 2020.

177. Ma, Y., A.J. Mouton, and M.L. Lindsey, *Cardiac macrophage biology in the steady-state heart, the aging heart, and following myocardial infarction.* Transl Res, 2018. **191**: p. 15-28.

178. Simoes, F.C., et al., *Macrophages directly contribute collagen to scar formation during zebrafish heart regeneration and mouse heart repair.* Nat Commun, 2020. **11**(1): p. 600.

179. Campisi, J. and L. Robert, *Cell senescence: role in aging and age-related diseases.* Interdiscip Top Gerontol, 2014. **39**: p. 45-61.

180. Childs, B.G., et al., *Cellular senescence in aging and age-related disease: from mechanisms to therapy.* Nat Med, 2015. **21**(12): p. 1424-35.

181. Gunawan, F., et al., *Nfatc1 Promotes Interstitial Cell Formation During Cardiac Valve Development in Zebrafish.* Circ Res, 2020. **126**(8): p. 968-984.

182. Benjamin, E.J., et al., *Heart Disease and Stroke Statistics-2019 Update: A Report From the American Heart Association.* Circulation, 2019. **139**(10): p. e56-e528.

183. Abdu, F.A., et al., *Effect of Secondary Prevention Medication on the Prognosis in Patients With Myocardial Infarction With Nonobstructive Coronary Artery Disease.* J Cardiovasc Pharmacol, 2020. **76**(6): p. 678-683.

184. Desai, P.A., J. Tafreshi, and R.G. Pai, *Beta-blocker therapy for valvular disorders.* J Heart Valve Dis, 2011. **20**(3): p. 241-53.

185. Antequera-Gonzalez, B., N. Martinez-Micaelo, and J.M. Alegret, *Bicuspid Aortic Valve and Endothelial Dysfunction: Current Evidence and Potential Therapeutic Targets.* Front Physiol, 2020. **11**: p. 1015.

186. van de Pol, V., et al., *Endothelial Colony Forming Cells as an Autologous Model to Study Endothelial Dysfunction in Patients with a Bicuspid Aortic Valve.* Int J Mol Sci, 2019. **20**(13).

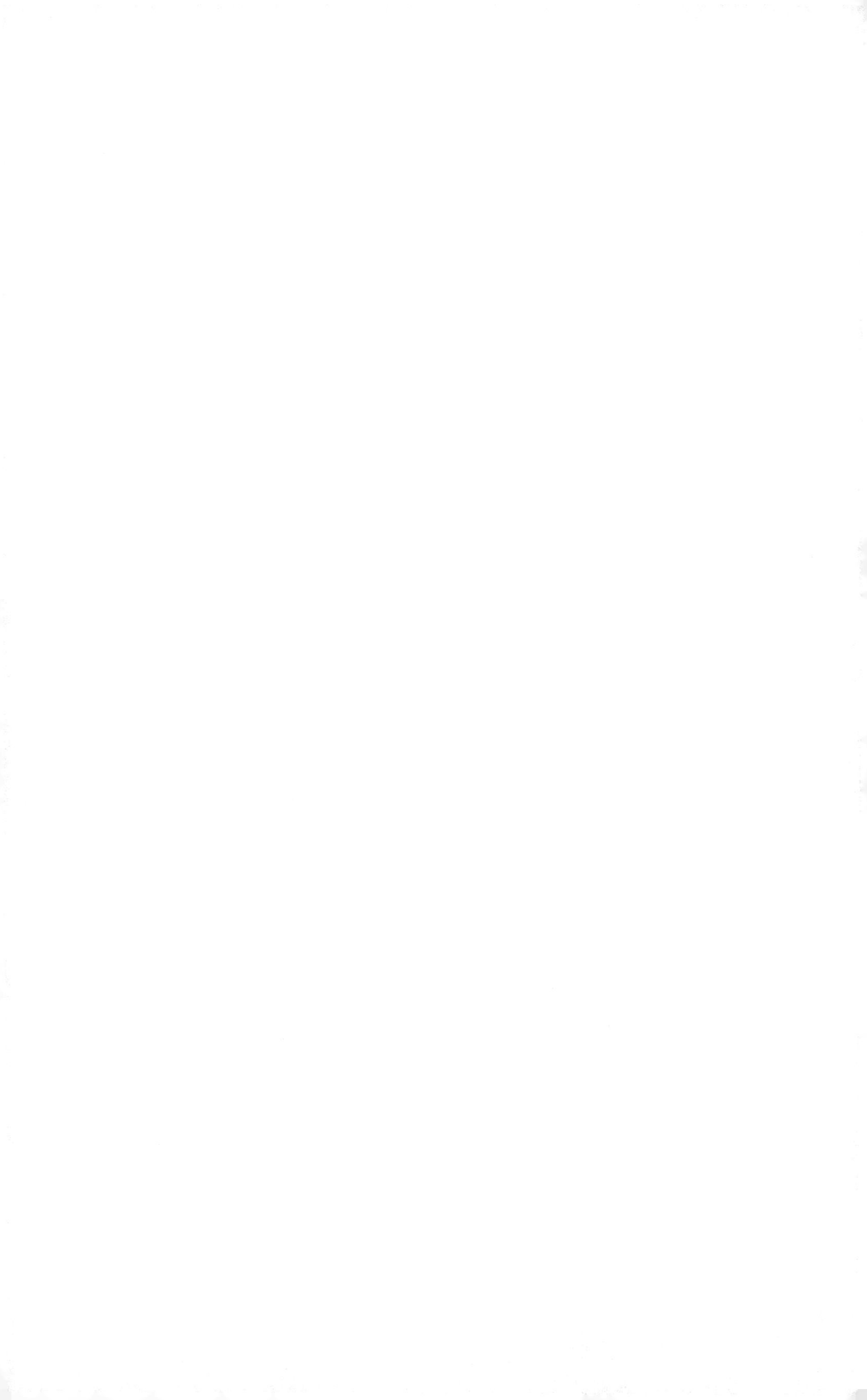